This report contains the collective views of an international group of experts and does not necessarily represent the decisions or the stated policy of the United Nations Environment Programme, the International Labour Organisation, or the World Health Organization.

Environmental Health Criteria 146

1,3-DICHLOROPROPENE, 1,2-DICHLOROPROPANE AND MIXTURES

Published under the joint sponsorship of the United Nations Environment Programme, the International Labour Organisation, and the World Health Organization

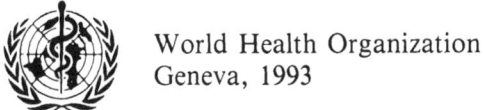

World Health Organization
Geneva, 1993

The **International Programme on Chemical Safety (IPCS)** is a joint venture of the United Nations Environment Programme, the International Labour Organisation, and the World Health Organization. The main objective of the IPCS is to carry out and disseminate evaluations of the effects of chemicals on human health and the quality of the environment. Supporting activities include the development of epidemiological, experimental laboratory, and risk-assessment methods that could produce internationally comparable results, and the development of manpower in the field of toxicology. Other activities carried out by the IPCS include the development of know-how for coping with chemical accidents, coordination of laboratory testing and epidemiological studies, and promotion of research on the mechanisms of the biological action of chemicals.

WHO Library Cataloguing in Publication Data

1,3-Dichloropropene, 1,2-dichloropropane and mixtures.

(Environmental health criteria ; 146)

1.Environmental exposure 2.Hydrocarbons, Chlorinated - adverse effects 3.Hydrocarbons, Chlorinated - poisoning 4.Hydrocarbons, Chlorinated - toxicity 5.Occupational exposure I.Series

ISBN 92 4 157146 2   (NLM Classification: QV 633)
ISSN 0250-8634

The World Health Organization welcomes requests for permission to reproduce or translate its publications, in part or in full. Applications and enquiries should be addressed to the Office of Publications, World Health Organization, Geneva, Switzerland, which will be glad to provide the latest information on any changes made to the text, plans for new editions, and reprints and translations already available.

©World Health Organization 1993

Publications of the World Health Organization enjoy copyright protection in accordance with the provisions of Protocol 2 of the Universal Copyright Convention. All rights reserved.

The designations employed and the presentation of the material in this publication do not imply the expression of any opinion whatsoever on the part of the Secretariat of the World Health Organization concerning the legal status of any country, territory, city or area or of its authorities, or concerning the delimitation of its frontiers or boundaries.

The mention of specific companies or of certain manufacturers' products does not imply that they are endorsed or recommended by the World Health Organization in preference to others of a similar nature that are not mentioned. Errors and omissions excepted, the names of proprietary products are distinguished by initial capital letters.

CONTENTS

ENVIRONMENTAL HEALTH CRITERIA FOR
1,3-DICHLOROPROPENE, 1,2-DICHLOROPROPANE,
AND MIXTURES

PART A. 1,3-DICHLOROPROPENE	9
PART B. 1,2-DICHLOROPROPANE	119
PART C. MIXTURES OF DICHLOROPROPENES AND DICHLOROPROPANE	163
REFERENCES	198
RESUME ET EVALUATION, CONCLUSIONS, ET RECOMMANDATIONS	223
RESUMEN Y EVALUACION, CONCLUSIONES, Y RECOMENDACIONES	243

WHO TASK GROUP ON ENVIRONMENTAL HEALTH CRITERIA FOR 1,3-DICHLOROPROPENE, 1,2-DICHLOROPROPANE, AND MIXTURES

Members

Dr V. Benes, Department of Toxicology and Reference Laboratory, Institute of Hygiene & Epidemiology, Prague, Czechoslovakia

Dr R. Drew, Key Centre for Toxicology, Department of Applied Biology, Royal Melbourne Institute for Technology, Melbourne, Victoria, Australia (*Chairman*)

Dr S.K. Kashyap, National Institute of Occupational Health, Ahmedabad, India

Dr J.I. Kundiev, Research Institute of Labour Hygiene & Occupational Diseases, Kiev, Ukraine (*Vice-Chairman*)

Dr K. Mitsumori, Division of Pathology, Biological Safety Research Center, National Institute of Hygienic Sciences, Tokyo, Japan

Dr Richard F. Shore, Ecotoxicology and Pollution Section, Institute of Terrestrial Ecology, Monks Wood Experimental Station, Abbots Ripton, Huntingdon, United Kingdom

Dr G.J. van Esch, Oranje, Bilthoven, Netherlands (*Rapporteur*)

Dr E.A.H. van Heemstra-Lequin, Laren, Netherlands (*Joint Rapporteur*)

Dr S. Wong, Bureau of Chemical Hazards, Environmental Health Directorate, Department of National Health and Welfare, Tunney's Pasture, Ottawa, Ontario, Canada

Observers

Dr D.E. Owen, Shell Internationale Petroleum Maatschappij BV, The Hague, Netherlands

Members from the Host Institution

- Dr W.H. Gross, Fraunhofer Institute of Toxicology & Aerosol Research, Hanover, Germany

- Dr J.R. Kielhorn, Fraunhofer Institute of Toxicology & Aerosol Research, Hanover, Germany

- Dr C.M. Melber, Fraunhofer Institute of Toxicology & Aerosol Research, Hanover, Germany

Secretariat

- Dr R.F. Hertel, Fraunhofer Institute of Toxicology & Aerosol Research, Hanover, Germany

- Dr K.W. Jager, International Programme on Chemical Safety, World Health Organization, Geneva, Switzerland (*Secretary*)

- Mme C. Partensky, Unit of Carcinogen Identification and Evaluation, International Agency for Research on Cancer (IARC), Lyon, France

NOTE TO READERS OF THE CRITERIA MONOGRAPHS

Every effort has been made to present information in the criteria monographs as accurately as possible without unduly delaying their publication. In the interest of all users of the Environmental Health Criteria monographs, readers are kindly requested to communicate any errors that may have occurred to the Director of the International Programme on Chemical Safety, World Health Organization, Geneva, Switzerland, in order that they may be included in corrigenda.

* * *

A detailed data profile and a legal file can be obtained from the International Register of Potentially Toxic Chemicals, Palais des Nations, 1211 Geneva 10, Switzerland (Telephone No. 7988400 or 7985850).

* * *

Note: The proprietary information contained in this monograph cannot replace documentation for registration purposes, because the latter has to be closely linked to the source, the manufacturing route, and the purity/impurities of the substance to be registered. The data should be used in accordance with paragraphs 82-84 and recommendations paragraph 90 of the Second FAO Government Consultation (1982).

ENVIRONMENTAL HEALTH CRITERIA FOR 1,3-DICHLOROPROPENE, 1,2-DICHLOROPROPANE, AND MIXTURES

The meeting of the WHO Task Group on Environmental Health Criteria for 1,3-dichloropropene, 1,2-dichloropropane, and mixtures, which was held at the Fraunhofer Institute of Toxicology and Aerosol Research, Hanover, Germany, from 16 to 20 September 1990, was sponsored by the German Ministry of the Environment. Dr R.F. Hertel welcomed the participants on behalf of the host institute. Dr K.W. Jager, IPCS, welcomed the participants on behalf of Dr M. Mercier, Director of the IPCS, and the three IPCS cooperating organizations (UNEP/ILO/WHO). The Group reviewed and revised the draft criteria monograph and made an evaluation of the risks for human health and the environment from exposure to 1,3-dichloropropene, 1,2-dichloropropane, and mixtures of dichloropropenes and dichloropropane.

Dr E.A.H. van Heemstra-Lequin and Dr G.J. van Esch of the Netherlands cooperated in the preparation of the first draft of the EHC monograph. Dr van Esch prepared the second draft, incorporating the comments received following circulation of the first draft to the IPCS contact points for Environmental Health Criteria monographs.

Dr K.W. Jager of the IPCS Central Unit was responsible for the scientific content of the monographs, and Mrs M.O. Head of Oxford for the editing.

The fact that Shell and Dow Chemical made their proprietary toxicological information on their products available to the IPCS and the Task Group is gratefully acknowledged. This allowed the Task Group to make their evaluation on a more complete data base.

The efforts of all who helped in the preparation and finalization of the publications are gratefully acknowledged.

* * *

Partial financial support for the publication of this criteria monograph was kindly provided by the United States Department of Health and Human Services, through a contract from the National Institute of Environmental Health Sciences, Research Triangle Park, North Carolina, USA - a WHO Collaborating Centre for Environmental Health Effects.

PART A

ENVIRONMENTAL HEALTH CRITERIA

FOR

1,3-DICHLOROPROPENE

CONTENTS

ENVIRONMENTAL HEALTH CRITERIA FOR
1,3-DICHLOROPROPENE

1. SUMMARY AND EVALUATION, CONCLUSIONS,
   AND RECOMMENDATIONS   15

   1.1 Summary and evaluation   15
       1.1.1 Use, environmental fate, and
              environmental levels   15
       1.1.2 Kinetics and metabolism   16
       1.1.3 Effects on organisms in the environment   17
       1.1.4 Effects on experimental animals and
              in vitro test systems   18
       1.1.5 Effects on human beings   21
   1.2 Conclusions   22
   1.3 Recommendations   22

2. IDENTITY, PHYSICAL AND CHEMICAL PROPERTIES,
   ANALYTICAL METHODS   24

   2.1 Identity   24
   2.2 Physical and chemical properties   25
   2.3 Conversion factors   26
   2.4 Analytical methods   26
       2.4.1 Sampling   26
       2.4.2 Determination of residues in crops and soil   30
       2.4.3 Determination of residues in water   31
       2.4.4 Determination of residues in air   31
       2.4.5 Determination of residues in food   32
       2.4.6 Determination of 3-chloroallyl alcohol   33
       2.4.7 Determination of mercapturic acids in urine   33

3. SOURCES OF HUMAN AND ENVIRONMENTAL
   EXPOSURE   35

   3.1 Natural occurrence   35
   3.2 Man-made sources   35
       3.2.1 Production levels and processes   35
       3.2.2 Use   36
       3.2.3 Sources of pollution   36

4. ENVIRONMENTAL TRANSPORT, DISTRIBUTION,
   AND TRANSFORMATION   37

	4.1	Transport and distribution between media	37
	4.1.1	Air	37
	4.1.2	Water	37
	4.1.3	Soil	39

        4.1 Transport and distribution between media   37
            4.1.1 Air   37
            4.1.2 Water   37
            4.1.3 Soil   39
                  4.1.3.1 Hydrolysis   40
                  4.1.3.2 Volatilization   44
                  4.1.3.3 Uptake in crops   45
                  4.1.3.4 Movement in soil   45
                  4.1.3.5 Loss under field conditions   46
                  4.1.3.6 Results of supervised field trials   49
        4.2 Bioconcentration   49
        4.3 Abiotic degradation   49
            4.3.1 Photodegradation   49
        4.4 Biodegradation and biotransformation   50
            4.4.1 Miscellaneous   53

5. ENVIRONMENTAL LEVELS AND HUMAN EXPOSURE   54

        5.1 Air   54
        5.2 Water   54
        5.3 Crops   56
        5.4 Occupational exposure   57

6. KINETICS AND METABOLISM   59

        6.1 Absorption, distribution, and elimination   59
            6.1.1 Oral   59
                  6.1.1.1 Rat   59
                  6.1.1.2 Mouse   60
            6.1.2 Inhalation   60
                  6.1.2.1 Rat   60
        6.2 Influence on tissue levels of glutathione   61
            6.2.1 Oral   61
            6.2.2 Inhalation   62
        6.3 Biotransformation   63
            6.3.1 Rat   63
            6.3.2 Humans   65
        6.4 Reaction with macromolecules   65
            6.4.1 Mouse   65
            6.4.2 Rat   66
        6.5 Appraisal   67

7. EFFECTS ON ORGANISMS IN THE ENVIRONMENT   68

        7.1 Acute toxicity   68

		7.1.1	Microorganisms	68
		7.1.2	Algae	69
		7.1.3	Invertebrates	70
		7.1.4	Honey bees	70
		7.1.5	Fish	71
		7.1.6	Birds	71
	7.2	Short-term/long-term toxicity		71
		7.2.1	Invertebrates	71
		7.2.2	Fish	74
		7.2.3	Field studies	74
		7.2.4	Phytotoxicity	74
8.	EFFECTS ON EXPERIMENTAL ANIMALS AND *IN VITRO* TEST SYSTEMS			75
	8.1	Single exposures		75
		8.1.1	Oral	75
		8.1.2	Inhalation	75
		8.1.3	Dermal	77
	8.2	Short-term exposures		79
		8.2.1	Oral	79
		8.2.2	Inhalation	79
			8.2.2.1 Mouse	79
			8.2.2.2 Rat	80
			8.2.2.3 Other animal species	83
	8.3	Skin and eye irritation, sensitization		83
		8.3.1	Skin irritation	83
		8.3.2	Eye irritation	84
			8.3.2.1 *In vitro* studies	85
		8.3.3	Sensitization	85
	8.4	Long-term exposure		86
	8.5	Reproduction, embryotoxicity, and teratogenicity		86
		8.5.1	Reproduction	86
			8.5.1.1 Inhalation (rat)	86
			8.5.1.2 Intraperitoneal (mouse)	87
		8.5.2	Teratogenicity	87
			8.5.2.1 Inhalation (rat)	87
			8.5.2.2 Inhalation (rabbit)	88
	8.6	Mutagenicity and related end-points		89
		8.6.1	*In vitro* studies	89
			8.6.1.1 Microorganisms	89
			8.6.1.2 Effects of glutathione on bacterial mutagenesis	93
			8.6.1.3 Mammalian cells	94
			8.6.1.4 DNA damage	94

			8.6.1.5 Chromosomal effects	95

        8.6.2 *In vivo* studies   96
        8.6.3 Appraisal   97
  8.7 Carcinogenicity   97
        8.7.1 Oral   97
                8.7.1.1 Mouse   97
                8.7.1.2 Rat   98
        8.7.2 Inhalation   100
                8.7.2.1 Mouse   100
                8.7.2.2 Rat   102
        8.7.3 Appraisal   104
        8.7.4 Dermal and subcutaneous (mouse)   106
  8.8 Factors modifying toxicity, toxicity of metabolites, mode of action   107
        8.8.1 Toxicity of metabolites, *cis*- and *trans*-1,3-dichloropropene oxide   107
                8.8.1.1 Mutagenicity   107
                8.8.1.2 Carcinogenicity   108
        8.8.2 Role of oxidation   108
        8.8.3 Role of glutathione   110
        8.8.4 Effect on liver enzyme activity   112

9. EFFECTS ON HUMANS   113

  9.1 General population   113
        9.1.1 Acute toxicity - poisoning incidents   113
        9.1.2 Controlled human studies   113
  9.2 Occupational exposure   114
        9.2.1 General   114
        9.2.2 Acute toxicity - poisoning incidents   116
        9.2.3 Effects of short- and long-term exposure   116

10. PREVIOUS EVALUATIONS BY INTERNATIONAL BODIES   117

1. SUMMARY AND EVALUATION, CONCLUSIONS, AND RECOMMENDATIONS

1.1 Summary and evaluation

1.1.1 Use, environmental fate, and environmental levels

"1,3-Dichloropropene" was introduced in 1956 as part of a mixture, containing 1,3-dichloropropenes, 1,2-dichloropropane, and other halogenated hydrocarbons, and has been widely used in agriculture as a pre-plant soil fumigant for the control of nematodes in vegetables, potatoes, and tobacco. Application is primarily by soil injection. The commercial formulation of 1,3-dichloropropene is a mixture of *cis*- and *trans*-isomers (in approximately equal proportions), which is a colourless to amber liquid with a penetrating, irritating, chloroform-like odour. The vapour pressure is 3.7 kPa at 20 °C. The technical product has a purity of 92% and may contain a number of impurities, such as 1,2-dichloropropane. The log P octanol/water partition coefficient is 1.98.

In air, decomposition of 1,3-dichloropropene is mainly by reaction with free radicals and ozone. The half-lives of the *cis*- and *trans*-isomers in the reaction with free radicals are 12 and 7 h, respectively, and in the reaction with ozone, 52 and 12 days, respectively. Direct photo-transformation seems to be insignificant, but may be enhanced in the presence of atmospheric particles.

In water, 1,3-dichloropropene is likely to disappear rapidly, because of its relatively low water solubility and high volatility; half-lives of less than 5 h have been reported.

The distribution of 1,3-dichloropropene in soil compartments is dependent on the vapour pressure, diffusion coefficient, temperature, and moisture content of the soil. The persistence of 1,3-dichloropropene in soil is influenced by volatilization, chemical and biological transformation, photochemical transformation, and organism uptake. Volatilization and diffusion in the vapour phase are the most significant mechanisms for environmental dispersion and dilution.

Transformation of 1,3-dichloropropene is initially by hydrolysis to 3-chloroallyl alcohol and then by microbial transformation to

3-chloroacrolein and 3-chloroacrylic acid. In a laboratory study, the half-lives for the hydrolysis of the *cis*- and *trans*-isomers of 1,3-dichloropropene at 15 °C and 29 °C were 11.0 and 2.0 days, respectively, for the *cis*-isomer and 13.0 and 2.0 days for the *trans*-isomer. In soil with a pH of 7 and a temperature of 25 °C, the half-life for hydrolysis for both isomers was 4.6 days. Because of its relatively rapid disappearance from soil, residues are unlikely to accumulate when the fumigant is applied at the recommended rate and frequency.

1,3-Dichloropropene is potentially mobile in soil, especially in open-textured, sandy soil with a low moisture content. Downward movement is enhanced by deep cultivation of soils with low porosity. 1,3-Dichloropropene has been detected in "upper groundwater" (up to 2 m below the surface), but not in deep groundwater, which is more likely to be used for drinking-water.

1,3-Dichloropropene can be taken up by crops. However, significant residues are unlikely to occur in edible crops, because these are not normally planted until most of the fumigant has dissipated.

Bioaccumulation of 1,3-dichloropropene is unlikely, because of its relatively high water solubility (> 1 g/kg), low log P octanol water partition coefficient, and rapid elimination from mammals and other organisms.

1.1.2 *Kinetics and metabolism*

1,3-Dichloropropene administered orally to rodents is rapidly eliminated. The major route of elimination is in the urine where 81% of the *cis*-isomer and 56% of the *trans*-isomer are eliminated within 24 h of dosing. The half-life of elimination in the urine is 5-6 h. Faecal elimination is minor. Expired carbon dioxide accounts for 4 and 24% of the elimination of the *cis*- and *trans*-isomers of 1,3-dichloropropene, respectively. Tissue concentrations after oral administration are low; the highest residual concentrations are found in the stomach wall, followed by lower amounts in the kidneys, liver, and bladder.

Unchanged 1,3-dichloropropene is not found in the urine. The *cis*- and *trans*-isomers are substrates for hepatic glutathione-*S*-alkyl transferase, forming mercapturic acids, which are excreted in the urine. The *trans*-isomer is conjugated 4-5 times more slowly than the *cis*-isomer. The principal urinary metabolite in rats and mice is N-acetyl-S-(3-chloroprop-2-enyl)L-cysteine; this compound can be used for biological monitoring in humans. A second, minor metabolic pathway has been identified for the *cis*-isomer that involves mono-oxygenation to *cis*-1,3-dichloropropene oxide, which can also be conjugated with glutathione. The high proportion of the *trans*-isomer that occurs in expired air results from an alternative metabolic pathway to conjugation that has a higher specificity for the *trans*- than for the *cis*-isomer.

Inhalation exposure of rats to 1,3-dichloropropene did not lead to increases in blood concentrations proportional with dose. At a dose of 408.6 mg/m^3 (90 ppm), respiratory frequency and respiratory minute volume were decreased and saturation of metabolism occurred at 1362 mg/m^3 (300 ppm). *Cis*- and *trans*-isomers were rapidly eliminated from the blood, the half-life of elimination being 3-6 min at concentrations below 1362 mg/m^3 but considerably longer (33-43 min) at higher concentrations.

1.1.3 Effects on organisms in the environment

The EC$_{50}$ values for growth (96 h) for the freshwater alga, *Selenastrum capricornutum*, and the estuarine diatom, *Skeletoneria costatum*, are 4.95 mg/litre and 1 mg/litre, respectively. The acute toxicity (96-h LC$_{50}$) of 1,3-dichloropropene for fish is of the order of 1-7.9 mg/litre. In an embryo-larval test on Fathead minnow, the maximum no-effect level was 0.24 mg/litre. These data and the fact that 1,3-dichloropropene is unlikely to persist in water, indicate that the hazard for fish lies in acute toxic effects, with little potential for additional effects resulting from long-term exposure.

1,3-dichloropropene at dose levels of 30-60 mg/kg can reduce the abundance of fungi and the rate of microbial enzyme activity, but the effect is not usually long lasting (< 7 days) and does not occur in all soil types. In some studies, there was a significant increase in microbial numbers following application.

1,3-Dichloropropene is phytotoxic, however, its toxicity for Honey bees is low. Using a dusting technique, the 48-h LD$_{50}$ was 6.6 µg/bee. Birds are relatively non-sensitive to 1,3-dichloropropene. LC$_{50}$s (8-day) of > 10 g/kg were reported for Mallard duck and Bobwhite quail.

1.1.4 Effects on experimental animals and in vitro test systems

The acute oral toxicity of 1,3-dichloropropene in animals is moderate to high. The LD_{50} values reported in rats ranged between 127 and 713 mg/kg body weight. The oral LD_{50} values in rats for the *cis*- and *trans*-isomers were 85 and 94 mg/kg body weight, respectively.

Acute dermal exposure is moderately toxic. Dermal LD_{50}s of 423 mg/kg body weight and 504 mg/kg body weight have been reported for the rat and the rabbit, respectively. The LD_{50} values for the *cis*- and *trans*-isomers were 1090 and 1575 mg/kg body weight, respectively.

Inhalation exposure (4 h) of rats indicated LC_{50}s of 3310 mg/m^3 (729 ppm) for 1,3-dichloropropene; 3042-3514 mg/m^3 for the *cis*-isomer, and 4880-5403 mg/m^3 for the *trans*-isomer.

Acute intoxication showed central nervous and respiratory system involvement.

Severe reactions were seen in rabbit skin and eye irritation tests, but recovery occurred in 14-21 days. The results of skin sensitization tests on guinea-pigs were positive.

Several short-term inhalation toxicity studies have been conducted on mice, rats, guinea-pigs, rabbits, and dogs. In mice, the nasal mucosa and urinary bladder were the target organs. Degeneration of the olfactory epithelium and hyperplasia of the respiratory epithelium were observed. Moderate hyperplasia of the transitional epithelium in the urinary bladder was found. A no-observed-effect level (NOEL) of 136 mg/m^3 (30 ppm) in mice can be estimated.

Similar degenerative changes of the olfactory epithelium and hyperplasia have been demonstrated in rats. The reported NOEL value for 1,3-dichloropropene from a well-designed study was 45.4 mg/m^3; a NOEL of 136 mg/m^3 has been reported for the *cis*-isomer.

A 90-day oral study on rats indicated a NOEL of 3 mg/kg body weight. The only observed effect at the next higher dose level of 10 mg/kg body weight was an increase in relative kidney weight in the male.

In a 2-generation, 2-litter, inhalation study on rats, doses of up to 408.6 mg/m^3 (90 ppm) did not show adverse effects on the reproduction parameters examined. However, the highest dose level of 408.6 mg/m^3 induced maternal toxicity, as evidenced by decreased growth and histopathological changes in the nasal mucosa. A NOEL of 136.2 mg/m^3 (30 ppm) was established for maternal toxicity.

Inhalation teratogenicity studies on rats and rabbits did not indicate teratogenic potential for 1,3-dichloropropene at exposure levels up to 1362 mg/m^3, but embryotoxicity (reduction in litter size and increase in resorption rates) was seen in the rat. Maternal toxicity was observed in both rats and rabbits at dose levels of 544.8 mg/m^3 (120 ppm) or more.

In most of the studies, *cis-* and *trans-*1,3-dichloropropene and mixtures were mutagenic in bacteria with, and without, metabolic activation. Pure 1,3-dichloropropene and pure *cis-*1,3-dichloropropene were found to be negative in bacteria. Glutathione was shown to prevent the mutagenic activity of 1,3-dichloropropene in bacteria. *Cis-*1,3-dichloropropene was negative in a gene mutation assay with V79 Chinese hamster cells as well as in the Chinese hamster ovary HPRT test.

Cis- and *trans-*1,3-dichloropropene induced unscheduled DNA synthesis in HeLa S$_3$ cells. In rat hepatocytes, 1,3-dichloropropene did not elicit significant DNA repair. 1,3-Dichloropropene was positive in the *Bacillus subtilis* strain H17 microsome rec-assay with metabolic activation.

In Chinese hamster ovary cells, *cis-* and *trans-*1,3-dichloropropene induced chromosome damage in the presence of metabolic activation but, in another study, 1,3-dichloropropene was positive without metabolic activation. *Cis-*1,3-dichloropropene did not induce chromosomal damage in rat liver cells, but induced sister chromatid exchange in Chinese hamster ovary cells with, and without, metabolic activation and in Chinese hamster V79 cells without activation.

1,3-Dichloropropene was negative in a bone marrow micronucleus test on mice and in a sex-linked, recessive lethal assay on *Drosophila melanogaster*.

Carcinogenicity studies were carried out on mice and rats. Technical 1,3-dichloropropene (containing 1% epichlorhydrin) was administered by gavage for 2 years. In mice, a significant increase in epithelial hyperplasia and transitional cell carcinomas in the urinary bladder, an increase in lung tumours, a slight increase in tumours of the liver, and an increase in epithelial hyperplasia and squamous cell papillomas or carcinomas in the forestomach were found. In rats, increases in the incidence of neoplastic nodules in the liver and of squamous cell papillomas or carcinomas of the forestomach were observed.

The carcinogenicity in mice and rats of 1,3-dichloropropene (without epichlorohydrin) was investigated in 2-year inhalation studies. In mice, increased incidences of hyperplasia of the urinary bladder, the forestomach, and the nasal mucosa were observed. There was an increase in the incidence of benign lung tumours. Some toxic changes in the olfactory mucosa of the nasal cavity were also seen in rats, but no increase in tumour incidence.

Epichlorohydrin was shown to produce forestomach tumours in a gavage study and nasal cavity tumours in an inhalation study on rats; a carcinogenic effect on the urinary bladder cannot be excluded for 1,3-dichloropropene administered orally to mice.

Mode of Action

Given that the major metabolic route of elimination of 1,3-dichloropropene is via conjugation with glutathione, it is to be expected that situations that affect tissue glutathione (non-protein sulfhydryl) concentrations may modify the effects of the compound. 1,3-Dichloropropene itself depletes the glutathione content of a variety of tissues, especially those that are the initial points of entry into the body, i.e., predominantly the forestomach and liver following gavage administration, and the nasal tissue after inhalation exposure. Decreases in nasal epithelium and forestomach glutathione occurred in mice after inhalation of 1,3-dichloropropene concentrations exceeding 22.7 mg/m^3 (5 ppm) and 113.5 mg/m^3 (25 ppm), respectively.

The toxicity of 1,3-dichloropropene in animals occurs at exposures that deplete glutathione and prior reduction of tissue glutathione exacerbates it. Long-term inhalation of concentrations higher than 90.8 mg/m^3 (20 ppm) results in degeneration and hyperplasia of nasal and stomach epithelia in mice, and long-term inhalation at 272.4 mg/m^3 (60 ppm) causes degeneration of nasal tissue in rats.

The protective role of glutathione has been further highlighted by studies demonstrating that covalent binding of ^{14}C-1,3-dichloropropene to mouse forestomach increased as the non-protein sulfhydryl content decreased. Similarly, in *in vitro* test systems, the genotoxicity of 1,3-dichloropropene and its minor oxidative (cytochrome P-450) metabolite (1,3-dichloropropene oxide) was markedly ameliorated by glutathione.

1.1.5 Effects on human beings

The exposure of the general population through air, water, or food is unlikely.

Studies have shown that occupational exposures are generally below 4.54 mg/m^3 (1 ppm), but higher levels have also been reported (up to 18.3 mg/m^3 during filling or nozzle changing). Occupational exposure is likely to be through inhalation and via the skin. Irritation of the eyes and the upper respiratory mucosa appears promptly after exposure. Inhalation of air containing concentrations of > 6810 mg/m^3 (> 1500 ppm) resulted in serious signs and symptoms of poisoning; lower exposures resulted in depression of the central nervous system and irritation of the respiratory system. Dermal exposure caused severe skin irritation.

Some liver and kidney function changes were reported in a group of 1,3-dichloroprepene applicators at the end of the application season. However, the cause-effect relationship has been contested.

Some poisoning incidents have occurred in which persons were hospitalized with signs and symptoms of irritation of the mucous membrane, chest discomfort, headache, nausea, vomiting, dizziness, and, occasionally, loss of consciousness and decreased libido. Three cases of haematological malignancies have been attributed to an earlier accidental overexposure to 1,3-dichloropropene, but the cause-effect relationship remains uncertain.

The fertility status of workers employed in the production of chlorinated three-carbon compounds was compared with a control group. There was no indication of an association between decreased fertility and exposure.

1.2 Conclusions

General population: In view of the low or non-existent exposure to 1,3-dichloropropene, the risk to the general population is negligible.

Occupational exposure: Filling operations and field applications may lead to operator exposure exceeding the maximum allowable concentration, when appropriate safety precautions have not been taken.

Environment: Provided that 1,3-dichloropropene is used at the recommended rate, it is unlikely to attain levels of environmental significance and is unlikely to have adverse effects on populations of terrestrial and aquatic organisms.

1.3 Recommendations

- Filling operations and field applications of 1,3-dichloropropene should only be conducted taking appropriate safety precautions, in order to ensure that exposure levels do not exceed the maximum allowable concentrations of 1,3-dichloropropene.

- Studies should be conducted to investigate the metabolic fate of *trans*-1,3-dichloropropene in mammals and the potential role that oxidative metabolites of this isomer may have in mediating 1,3-dichloropropene toxicity.

- Glutathione transferase mediates the protective effect of glutathione against the toxicity of 1,3-dichloropropene. It is recommended that studies should be carried out to compare the relative enzyme kinetics of human glutathione S-transferase from various tissues with enzyme activity from comparable animal tissues.

- The available data on the protective role of glutathione should be consolidated and published in the open literature.

- Part of the genotoxicity of dichloropropene is mediated by oxidative metabolism. It is recommended that studies be undertaken to identify the responsible cytochrome P-450 isoenzyme and compare its activity with human P-450 isoenzymes.

- The confounding role of epichlorohydrin in oral gavage carcinogenicity studies should be clarified.

2. IDENTITY, PHYSICAL AND CHEMICAL PROPERTIES, ANALYTICAL METHODS

2.1 Identity

Primary constituents

Chemical structure

```
ClCH₂       Cl        ClCH₂       H
     \    /                \    /
      C=C                   C=C
     /    \                /    \
    H      H              H      Cl
       (Z)                   (E)
```

Cis or (Z)1,3-dichloropropene   Trans or (E)1,3-dichloropropene

Chemical formula	$C_3H_4Cl_2$
Relative molecular mass	110.98
Chemical name	1,3-dichloropropene; (IUPAC); dichloro-1,3-propene; (F-ISO); 1,3-dichloro-1-propene; (CA).
Common synonyms	γ-chloroallylchloride, 1,3-dichloropropylene
Trade name	TELONE II®, D-D 92
CAS registry number	542-75-6 (*cis*- and *trans*-isomers) *cis*-isomer: 10061-01-5 *trans*-isomer: 10061-02-6
RTECS registry number	UC8310000
EINECS number	208-826-5

The commercial product is a mixture of *cis*- and *trans*-isomers and is more than 92% pure. In the past, 1% epichlorohydrin was added as a stabilizer, but nowadays an epoxidized vegetable oil is used.

Other names are: Dedisol C, Nematox II, D-D 95, Telone 2000 (Hayes, 1982; Worthing & Hance, 1991).

.2 Physical and chemical properties

Freezing point	- 85 °C[a] (*cis*-isomer)
Boiling point	103.8-105.2 °C (*cis*-isomer)[a] 111.0-112.0 °C (*trans*-isomer)[b] 108.0 °C (1,3-dichloropropene)
Vapour pressure at 25 °C	4850 Pa (*cis*-isomer)[a] 3560 Pa (*trans*-isomer)[b] 3.7 kPa (20 °C) (1,3-dichloropropene)
Relative density (D 23/4) (D 20/4)	1.221 kg/litre (*cis*-isomer)[a] 1.214 kg/litre (*trans*-isomer)[b]
Water solubility (at 20 °C, in g/litre)	2.45 (*cis*-isomer)[a] 2.49 (*trans*-isomer)[b] 2.0 (1,3-dichloropropene)
Flash point	28.5 °C (*cis*-isomer)[a] 28.0 °C (*trans*-isomer)[b] 25.0 °C (1,3-dichloropropene)
Self-ignition	555 °C (*cis*-isomer)[a] 534 °C (*trans*-isomer)[b]
Log P octanol/water partition coefficient	1.82 at 20 °C (*cis*-isomer)[a] 2.22 at 25 °C (*trans*-isomer)[b] 1.4-2.0 (1,3-dichloropropene)
K(OM/V[c]	14 (*cis*-isomer) 15 (*trans*-isomer)
K (OM/V)[c]	14 (*cis*-isomer) 15 (*trans*-isomer)

[a] purity 98.1%;
[b] purity 96.7%;
[c] K(OM/V) = μg adsorbed per g of organic matter (soil)
             μg dissolved per ml water phase

From: Leistra (1970), Krijgsheld & van der Gen (1986), Bennett & Ridge (1989), Schuurman (1989), van Hooidonk (1989), O'Connor (1990a).

Neither the *cis*- nor the *trans*-isomer produces gas in contact with water, and they are not highly flammable in contact with diatomite.

1,3-Dichloropropene is a colourless to amber coloured liquid with a penetrating, irritating, chloroform-like odour. The technical product is > 92% pure. The physical properties of a *cis/trans* mixture depend on the ratio of the isomers (Yang, 1986).

Saturated atmosphere: 167 980 mg/m^3 (37 000 ppm) at 25 °C. Explosive limit: 195 220 mg/m^3 (43 000 ppm) (80 °C). Miscible with acetone, benzene, carbon tetrachloride, heptane, and methanol (Sittig, 1980; Hayes, 1982; Worthing & Hance, 1991).

Van Hooidonk (1989) and O'Connor (1990a) described methods to determine the water- and/or fat solubility of *cis*- and *trans*-1,3-dichloropropene using gas chromatography and ECD and/or FID detection.

Details on ultraviolet/visible, infrared, and nuclear magnetic resonance spectra are given by O'Connor (1990a).

2.3 Conversion factors

1 ppm (91.2% 1,3-dichloropropene) = 4.54 mg/m^3 at 25 °C at 1 atm (Krijgsheld & Van der Gen, 1986; Breslin et al., 1987).

2.4 Analytical methods

Methods have been developed for the determination of 1,3-dichloropropene (*cis*- and *trans*-isomers) and of 1,2-dichloropropane in air, soil, water, and crops, and the degradation product 3-chloroallyl alcohol (*cis*- and *trans*-isomers) in soil and crops (see Tables 1 and 2). Current methods are based on gas chromatography (GC).

2.4.1 Sampling

In the case of crops and soil, the need for special care in the handling of samples and extracts has been stressed, because of the high volatility of 1,3-dichloropropene.

To minimize loss of residue by volatilization, soil samples should be deep frozen as soon as possible after sampling, and shipped to the laboratory for analysis in sealed containers with a

Table 1. Methods of analysis for 1,3-dichloropropene and 1,2-dichloropropane in food and biological media

Sample	Extraction	Clean-up	Detection and quantitation	Recovery	Limit of determination	Reference
Crops, Soil	steam distillation and diethyl ether extraction	absorption chromatography on acidic alumina	gas chromatography with ECD and FID	-[a]	0.01 mg/kg (1,3-dichloropropene) 0.1 mg/kg (1,2-dichloropropane)	Rexilius & Schmidt (1982); Shell (1985); Wallace (1974)
	trapped in ethyl acetate	-	gas chromatography with ECD	-[a]	-	Shell (1980)
Water	steam distillation and diethyl ether extraction	absorption chromatography on acidic alumina	gas chromatography with ECD	-[a]	0.001 mg/kg (1,2-dichloropropane)	Shell (1985)
Air	-	absorption on Tenax GC, desorption with isooctane	gas chromatography with ECD	-[a]	-[a]	Leiber & Berk (1984)

Table 1 (contd).

Sample	Extraction	Clean-up	Detection and quantitation	Recovery	Limit of determination	Reference
Air	-	absorption on charcoal, desorption with carbon disulfide	gas chromatography with FID	90-100%	0.005 mg/m^3	Van Sittert et al. (1977); Sherren & Woodbridge (1987a,b)
Air	-	absorption on charcoal, desorption with methanol/benzene	gas chromatography with ECD	85%	23 ng[b]	Albrecht et al. (1986)
Blood	hexane	-	gas chromatography with ^{63}Ni-ECD or GS-MS (SIM)	90%	cis and trans 1,3-dichloropropene, 5.3-5.9 ng/litre	Kastl & Hermann (1983)

[a] Data on recovery and/or limit of determination not given.
[b] Given as mass/tube.

Table 2. Methods of analysis for 3-chloroallyl alcohol in food and biological media

Sample	Extraction	Clean-up	Detection and quantitation	Recovery	Limit of determination	Reference
Crop, Soil	diethyl ether	derivatization with 3,5-dinitrobenzoyl chloride and pyridine, absorption chromatography on acidic alumina	gas chromatography with ECD	-	crops: 0.05 mg/kg soil: 0.02 mg/kg	Rexilius & Schmidt (1982) Wallace (1974)
Crop, Soil, Water	steam-distillation, hexane extraction with diethyl ether	esterification with trifluoroacetic anhydride	capillary gas-chromatography with ECD	- - -	- - water: 0.002 mg/kg	Shell (1978) Shell (1985)

minimum of delay (Rexilius & Schmidt, 1982). The period of storage of deep frozen samples in the laboratory should also be kept as short as possible (Wallace, 1979). At -20 °C, Hermann & Matsuyama (1982) found a slow decline in the contents of all components of "MIX D/D", indicating a maximum acceptable storage period of 2 months. No loss occurred in 4 months at a temperature of -80 °C.

Crop samples should be deep frozen as soon as possible after sampling, and water samples should be chilled or deep frozen; both should be shipped and stored under the same precautions as soil (Wallace, 1976b; Rexilius & Schmidt, 1982).

2.4.2 Determination of residues in crops and soil

A combined method for the determination and confirmation of 1,3-dichloropropene, 1,2-dichloropropane, and chloroallyl alcohol (3-CAA) in crops and soil has been developed (Wallace, 1974; Shell, 1976). After steam distillation and extraction and clean up, the determination of residues is carried out using gas chromatography (electron capture (ECD) and flame ionization (FID)). The chloroallyl alcohol is derivatized, followed by a clean up and determination using ECD. Confirmation of the identity of residues is carried out by combined gas chromatography-mass spectrometry (GC-MS).

With this method, the lower limit of determination in most crop and soil samples is 0.01 mg/kg for 1,3-dichloropropene and 0.1 mg/kg for 1,2-dichloropropane. For 3-chloroallyl alcohol, the lower limit of determination is 0.05 mg/kg for crops and 0.02 mg/kg for soil (Wallace, 1974; Rexilius & Schmidt, 1982; Shell, 1985).

Alternative methods are described by Shell (1980) in which 1,3-dichloropropene and 1,2-dichloropropane are trapped in ethyl acetate and directly determined, without clean up by capillary GC with ECD. The 3-chloroallyl alcohol residues are steam-distilled without acid or alkali and "free residues" are washed with hexane, and extracted into diethyl ether. The alcohol residues are then esterified by trifluoroacetic anhydride and determined with capillary GC with ECD (Shell, 1978).

Shell (1984) described a method based on the previously mentioned techniques of extraction and preparation of extracts; however, in both crops and soil, residues are determined by capillary GC with a Hall electrolytic conductivity detector (HECD). In addition, residues of 3-chloroallyl alcohol are determined without derivatization. The lower limit of determination is 0.01 mg/kg.

2.4.3 Determination of residues in water

The methods described in section 2.4.2 can be adapted for the determination of residues of 1,3-dichloropropene, 1,2-dichloropropane, and 3-chloroallyl alcohol in water (Wallace, 1974). The alternative methods mentioned under section 2.4.2 also include procedures for water analysis (Wallace, 1974; Shell, 1978) (see Table 1).

A laboratory analytical method (US EPA method 524.2), developed to monitor drinking-water, involves a standard inert (helium) gas purge extraction, isolation on a solid-phase trap (gas chromatography with a fused silica capillary column (FSCC) coated with a film of cyanopropylphenyl-dimethylpolysiloxane polymer), thermal desorption, and gas chromatography and identification and measurement with a low-cost, bench-top ion trap detector (ITD), which functions as a mass spectrometer. At a concentration of 0.2 µg/litre, the total mean measurement accuracy was 99% for *trans*-1.3-dichloropropene (*cis*-isomer not measured) and 103% for 1,2-dichloropropane (Eichelberger et al., 1990).

Telliard (1990) described broad-range methods for the determination of pollutants in waste water. US EPA method 1624 is used to determine purgeable organic compounds by calibrated isotope dilution or internal standard GC-MS and by reverse search of a GS-MS run for the analytes. The first technique can be used to determine 1,2-dichloropropane and the second, 1,3-dichloropropene.

2.4.4 Determination of residues in air

Methods based on the use of solid absorbent traps or direct gas sampling procedures in conjunction with GC analysis have been described for the determination of 1,3-dichloropropenes and 1,2-dichloropropane in air.

Leiber & Berk (1984) used Tenax-GC as an absorbent to monitor concentrations of chlorinated aliphatic hydrocarbons in workspace air. Isooctane, containing 1,3,5-tribromobenzene as internal standard, was used for the desorption of the hydrocarbons. Recoveries of 1,3-dichloropropenes were in the range of 1.8-18 mg/m^3. A similar method was used by Van Sittert et al. (1977) and Albrecht et al. (1986), but, in this case, the trapping medium was activated charcoal. It appears that charcoal had a better trapping capacity than Tenax-GC (Brown & Purnell, 1979) for 1,3-dichloropropenes. Trapped vapours were desorbed using carbon disulfide (recovery 90-100%) (van Sittert et al., 1977; HSE, 1990) or 1% v/v methanol-benzene mixture (mean recovery 85%) (Albrecht et al., 1986). Van Sittert et al. (1977) could determine 0.05 mg/m^3 of the *cis*- and *trans*-isomers of 1,3-dichloropropene in air.

All authors warned that care should be taken in the handling of trapped samples.

Parker et al. (1982) used charcoal filters to determine 1,3-dichloropropene and 1,2-dichloropropane levels in air.

Others have used more direct gas sampling procedures. Air from the head space above soil and water in sealed containers has been sampled and directly determined by GC with ECD or FID. Gas samples were trapped by injecting the air into an organic solvent, such as xylene or hexane, before GC analysis (Williams, 1968; Leistra, 1970; Abdalla, 1974; Abdalla et al., 1974; McKenry & Thomason, 1974; van Dijk, 1980).

2.4.5 Determination of residues in food

Reinert et al. (1983) described a dynamic heated headspace analysis of organic compounds including 1,2-dichloropropane in fish and shellfish tissue samples. The method included solvent (carbon disulfide) desorption of activated carbon adsorbent and determination with capillary column gas chromatography with a flame ionization detector. Recoveries were rather low (approximately 40-70%). Hiatt (1983) described a vacuum distillation apparatus and a procedure developed for the analysis of fish tissue. The volatile compounds were distilled from the sample and characterized by gas chromatography/mass spectrometry using fused silica capillary column (FSCC).

A method was described by Daft (1989) to determine fumigants and related chemicals in fatty and non-fatty foods. The method started with liquid extraction with isooctane, when necessary with co-extraction with a mixture of acetone/NaCl in 25% phosphoric acid and isooctane. The isooctane extracts were analysed using gas chromatography. Excess fat was removed by micro-Florisil columns. The determination was done by ECD and HECD (Hall electroconductivity detection). Overall mean recovery was 73% from fatty foods and 78% from non-fatty foods; the recovery from both sample types after further Florisil chromatography was 55%.

2.4.6 Determination of 3-chloroallyl alcohol

In Table 2, analytical methods are described to determine 3-chloroallyl alcohol in food and biological media.

2.4.7 Determination of mercapturic acids in urine

In Table 3, methods are described to determine metabolites of 1,3-dichloropropene in urine.

Van Welie et al. (1989) used an analytical method to determine N-acetyl-S-(cis- and trans)-3-chloroprop-2-enyl-L-cysteine (cis- and trans-DCP-MA) in urine, based on capillary gas chromatography with sulfur-selective detection. An internal standard N-acetyl-S-(benzyl)-L-cysteine and hydrochloric acid (resulting in a pH 1-2) were added to urine samples. The samples were extracted with ethyl acetate and the latter evaporated; the residues were methylated and determined using gas chromatography-flame photometric detection (GC-FPD). GC-MS was used for identification. The limits of determination were 0.107 mg/litre for cis-DCP-MA and 0.115 mg/litre for trans-DCP-MA.

Table 3. Methods of analysis for metabolites of 1,3-dichloropropene in urine

Sample	Extraction derivatization	Clean-up derivatization	Detection and quantitation	Recovery	Limit of determination	Reference
N-acetyl-S[cis-chloroprop-2-enyl]cysteine						
Urine (human)	ether	derivatization with diazomethane etherate	gas chromatography with electron impact ionization silicone membrane separator, mass spectrometry	-	-	Osterloh et al. (1984)
Urine (human)	ethyl acetate	derivatization with diazomethane etherate	gas chromatography with fused silica WCOT columns, sulfur-selective detection	*cis*-isomer and *trans*-isomer 105%	for *cis*- and *trans*-isomer range 107-115 ng/ml	van Welie et al. (1989)
Urine (rat)	ethyl acetate	derivatization with diazomethane	gas chromatography with nitrogen selective detection or negative chemical ionization/mass spectrometry	*cis*-isomer 66-83% *trans*-isomer 56-85%	for the different methods and for *cis*- and *trans*-isomer range 20-550 ng/ml	Onkenhout et al. (1986)

3. SOURCES OF HUMAN AND ENVIRONMENTAL EXPOSURE

3.1 Natural occurrence

As far as is known, 1,3-dichloropropene does not occur naturally.

3.2 Man-made sources

3.2.1 Production levels and processes

1,3-Dichloropropene is produced by the high-temperature chlorination of propylene or from 1,3-dichloro-2-propanol by dehydration with $POCl_3$ or with P_2O_5 in benzene.

1,3-Dichloropropene is a by-product in the synthesis of allyl chloride; 1,2-dichloropropane and to a lesser extent, 2,3-dichloropropene are also formed. In some commercial products, marketed for soil fumigation (mix D/D, Telone), 1,3-dichloropropene is the major and active ingredient (50-80% of total), but 1,2-dichloropropane (20-40%) and 2,3-dichloropropene (5-6.5%) are also present (Krijsheld & Van der Gen, 1986).

Before 1978, about 25 000 tonnes of 1,3-dichloropropene were produced annually in the USA (Flessel et al., 1978). In Italy, 2187 tonnes were produced in 1972 (De Lorenzo et al., 1977). Over 1285 tonnes of 1,3-dichloropropene-containing pesticides were used in California in 1971 (Yang, 1986), while in the period 1970-77, the amount applied was approximately 1.8-2.7 million kg. In 1981, over 7.2 million kg of 1,2-dichloropropane- and 1,3-dichloropropene-containing fumigants were used in California (California State Water Resources Control Board, 1983).

The estimated production in Europe in 1979 was 6-7 kilotonnes/year.

1,2-Dichloropropane, present as an impurity in the fumigant, does not add to the desired biological effects, but may, on the contrary, have unwanted ecotoxicological consequences. Therefore, there has been a more recent development to stop the use of the "impure" fumigant and to move to a purer preparation of 1,3-dichloropropene (> 90%) (Krijsheld & Van der Gen, 1986).

3.2.2 Use

1,3-Dichloropropene, the main ingredient of Telone II, was introduced in 1956 as a commercial preplant soil fumigant for the control of nematodes in crops, such as vegetables, potatoes, and tobacco. It is applied from a tractor-drawn, high pressure injection system into the soil. The soil is treated prior to the planting of crops (De Lorenzo et al., 1977; Hayes, 1982; Maddy et al., 1982).

1,3-Dichloropropene is effective against soil nematodes including root-knot, meadow, sting and dagger, spiral and sugar beet nematodes. The rates of application are determined according to the crop to be grown and the soil conditions, but generally lie within the range of 75-200 kg/ha (occasional maximum of 700 kg/ha) (Krijgsheld & van der Gen, 1986; Shell, IPM, 1990).

3.2.3 Sources of pollution

1,3-Dichloropropene is used extensively as a soil fumigant for the treatment of agricultural land. After application, part of the chemical will evaporate and escape from the soil. Although significant biodegradation and abiotic decomposition will occur in the soil, there is a limited risk of leaching down to groundwater level (see section 4.1.3). The 1,3-dichloropropene that is used for fumigation is contaminated with 1,2-dichloropropane and 2,3-dichloropropene. At application rates of "MIX D/D" ranging from 200 to 400 kg/ha, this may mean an input of 40-160 kg of 1,2-dichloropropane and 10-25 kg of 2,3-dichloropropene per hectare of land (Krijgsheld & van der Gen, 1986). The potential for groundwater contamination has been reduced by reducing the 1,2-dichloropropane content of the products used in agriculture.

4. ENVIRONMENTAL TRANSPORT, DISTRIBUTION, AND TRANSFORMATION

As with other fumigants, the performance of 1,3-dichloropropene as a nematocide is dependent on a number of important factors influencing the movement of soil fumigants, e.g., the chemical and adsorptive characteristics of the toxicant (vapour pressure, solubility, diffusion coefficient, the distribution of the fumigant through air, water, and solid phases of the soil) and physical factors, such as temperature, moisture, organic matter, soil texture, and soil profile variability (Munnecke & van Gundy, 1979; NTP, 1985; Yang, 1986).

Dichloropropenes can enter the aquatic environment as discharges from industrial effluents, through run off from agricultural land, and from municipal effluents.

The stability and mobility of 1,3-dichloropropene and 1,2-dichloropropane in air, soil, and groundwater are influenced by several processes, as shown in Fig. 1.

4.1 Transport and distribution between media

(See also section 4.1 of 1,2-dichloropropane and subsections).

4.1.1 Air

Tuazon et al. (1984) calculated that, at a daytime OH-radical concentration of $2 \times 10^6/cm^3$ (8×10^{-8} ppm) in the troposphere, the half-lives of *cis-* and *trans-*1,3-dichloropropene would be 12 and 7 h, respectively. The half-life for 1,2-dichloropropane is ≥ 313 days for a 24-h average OH-radical concentration of $1 \times 10^6/cm^3$. For the reaction with ozone at a background level in the troposphere of 80 $\mu g/m^3$ (0.04 ppm), the half-lives of *cis-* and *trans-*1,3 dichloropropene, were calculated to be 52 and 12 days. Direct phototransformation seems to be insignificant compared with the two other reactions, but may be enhanced in the presence of atmospheric particulates.

4.1.2 Water

Since the chloropropenes have a relatively low water solubility and high volatility, they will have a tendency to disappear rapidly from an aqueous medium. The half-life of evaporation of a

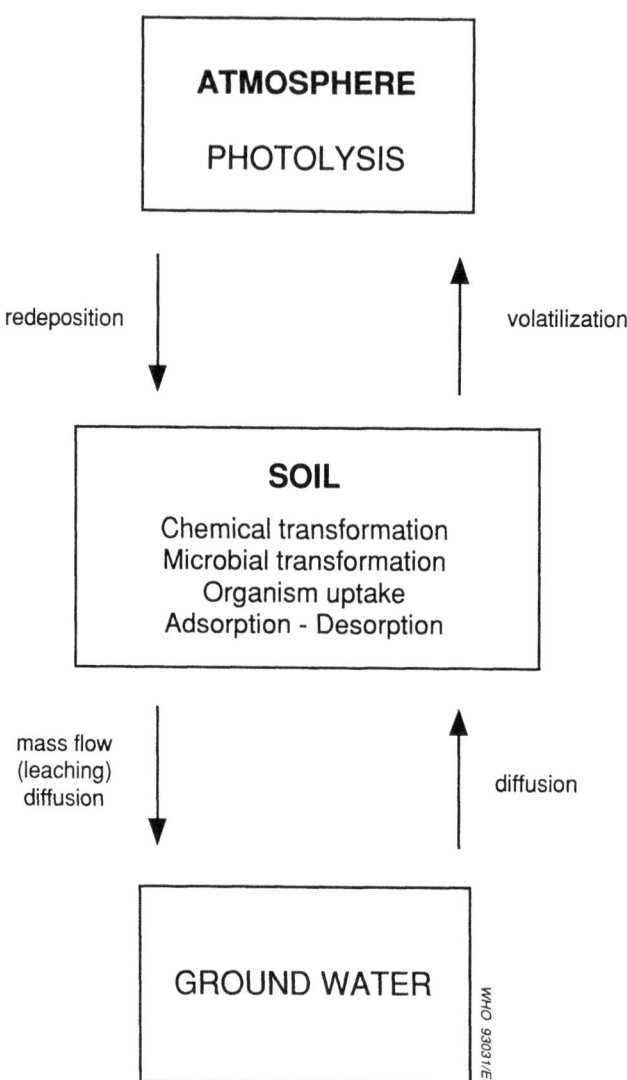

Fig. 1. Environmental fate of 1,3-dichloropropene and 1,2-dichloropropane. From: California State Water Resources Control Board (1983).

chemical from a certain body of water will increase with the depth of the water and continuous evaporation will become increasingly dependent on sufficient agitation in the water. Evaporation can be expected to contribute significantly to the disappearance from the aquatic environment (Krijgsheld & van der Gen, 1986).

Dilling et al. (1975) determined the rate of evaporation of 1,3-dichloropropene (*cis*- and *trans*-) from water at the 1 mg/litre level under ambient conditions. The time required for the compound to be reduced by 50% was 31 min and by 90%, 98 min.

Yon et al. (1991) determined that the half-life of evaporation of 1,3-dichloropropene (*cis*- and *trans*-isomers) from water was less than 5 h.

4.1.3 Soil

The persistence of 1,3-dichloropropene depends on chemical degradation, volatilization, microbial transformation, photochemical transformation, type of soil, water content of soil, and uptake into organisms. Thomason & McKenry (1974) studied the quantitative as well as the qualitative aspects of the movement and fate of 1,3-dichloropropene under various conditions in different types of soil.

Since 1,3-dichloropropene is used as soil fumigant, some information is available on the distribution of the compound in soil. The adsorption of 1,3-DCP on soil was found to be proportional to the organic matter content of the soil. The $K(om/v)s$[a] for *cis*- and *trans*-1,3-dichloropropene were estimated to be 14 and 15, respectively, independent of ambient temperature (Leistra, 1970). Similar soil/water distribution coefficients (23 and 26), based on organic carbon content, were reported by Kenaga (1980).

McKenry & Thomason (1974) demonstrated that high soil moisture was a major limiting factor in the total diffusion when soil moisture in the field approached field capacity. In contrast, Munnecke & van Gundy (1979) stated that soil moisture was a very important factor in that gaseous compounds are most

---

[a] See section 2.2.

effective in killing organisms when they are in a moist environment.

Environmental transformation of 1,3-dichloropropene results from microbial action, with the exception of the initial hydrolysis of *cis*- and *trans*-1,3-dichloropropene to 3-chloroallyl alcohol (Castro & Belser, 1966; Belser & Castro, 1971). The pathway for the transformation of 1,3-dichloropropene is given in Fig. 2.

4.1.3.1 Hydrolysis

Cis- and *trans*-1,3-dichloropropene can be hydrolysed in soil to 3-chloroallyl alcohol (see Fig. 2). Hydrolysis rates for 1,3-dichloropropenes range from 1 to 3.4% per day, depending on temperature and moisture content. Hydrolysis rates also vary with soil type (particle size) because of differences in chemical diffusion rate and sorption capacity (California State Water Resources Control Board, 1983).

Using [^{14}C]-radiolabelled 1.3-dichloropropene in sterile buffered water at pH 5, 7, or 9 and temperatures of 10, 20, or 30 °C, McCall (1987) found that the rate of hydrolysis was independent of pH at each temperature, and that the half-lives at temperatures of 30, 20, and 10 °C were 3.1, 11.3, and 51 days, respectively. One hydrolysis product, formed during the course of the study, was identified as 3-chloroallyl alcohol. The alcohol appeared to be stable to further hydrolytic conversion and was formed in the same *cis*-:*trans*-ratio as the initial 1,3-dichloropropene.

The hydrolysis of *cis*-1,3-dichloropropene (98.1%) was studied by O'Connor (1990b). The degradation reactions at all pH values were shown to follow pseudo first-order behaviour in the EEC-test, independent of the concentration. The degradation rate constants and environmental half-lives for *cis*-1,3-dichloropropene at 25 °C at pH 4, pH 7, and pH 9 (extrapolated by measuring degradation at temperatures of 50, 60, and 70 °C, using Arrhenius relationships) were 100 h, 54.5 h, and 38 h, respectively. (Remark: although the rate of hydrolysis of *cis*-1,3-dichloropropene did show some slight pH dependence, the author stated that this was probably within experimental error). It is hypothesized that the degradation proceeds via a resonance stabilized carbonium ion intermediate, resulting in the formation of a mixture of 3-chloroallyl alcohol and propenal (see Fig. 3).

1,3-Dichloropropene

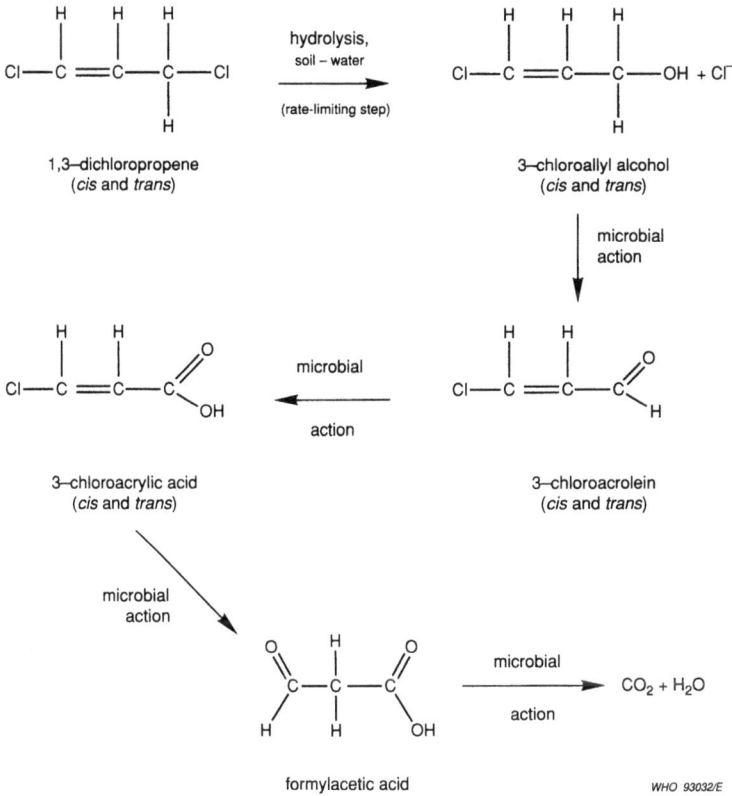

Fig. 2. Environmental transformation of 1,3-dichloropropene
Adapted from: California State Water Resources Control Board (1983),
Roberts & Stoydin (1976), van Dijk (1974), Belser & Castro (1971), and Perry & Roberts (1974).

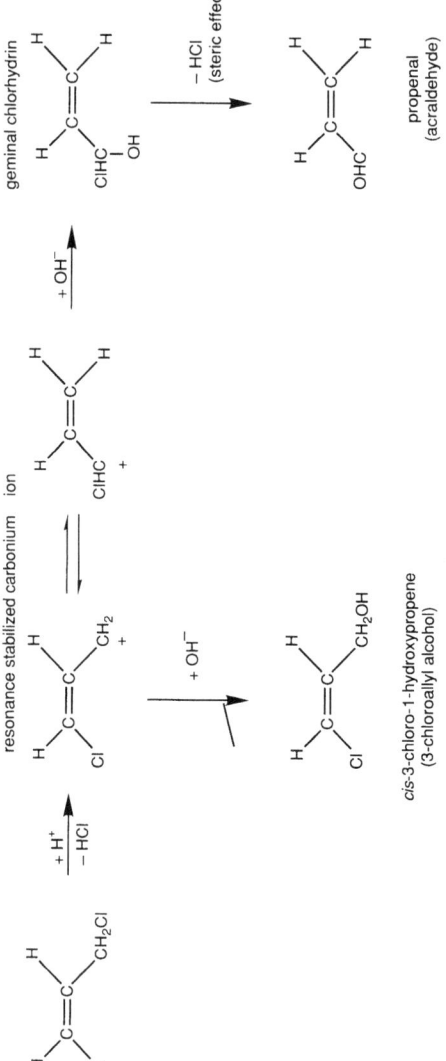

Fig. 3. Proposed reaction mechanism for the acid and base hydrolyses of cis-1,3-dichloropropene. SN1 mechanism (acid/base promoted via resonance stabilized carbonium ion intermediate). From: O'Connor (1990b).

Connors et al. (1990) studied the hydrolysis of 1,3-dichloropropene into 3-chloroallyl alcohol, under laboratory conditions. A 1.0 µg/litre *cis*- and *trans*-1,3-dichloropropene solution was prepared in a pH 5.5 or pH 7.0 buffer. The half-lives for the *cis*- and *trans*-isomers at 15 and 29 °C (pH 5.5) were 11.0, 2.0 and 13.0, 2.0 days, respectively. At pH 7.0 and 25 °C, the value was 4.6 days for both isomers.

Determination of the rate of hydrolysis of 1,3-dichloropropene at 25 °C in 50% aqueous ethanol indicated a half-time of 4 days for both the *cis*- and *trans*-isomers and appeared independent of the concentration in the range of 10-1000 mg/litre. Only small differences were observed in disappearance rates at pH levels of 5.5 and 7.5. The effect of temperature was clearly demonstrated: at 29 °C, the half-life for *cis*-1,3-dichloropropene was 1.5-2.0 days, while, at 2 °C, the half-life was estimated to be 91-100 days (Krijgsheld & Van der Gen, 1986).

The rates of transformation of the *cis*- and *trans*-isomers in soil layers of 0.1-0.2 m and 0.4-0.5 m in a bulb field in the Netherlands were determined in the laboratory. The initial contents of added 1,3-dichloropropene were approximately 12 and 62 mg/kg. Incubation took place at 15 °C. The half transformation time was about 4 days for both isomers. After 2 weeks, only small amounts (1%) of the initial amount were left. The transformation was slower in soil with the higher initial content (62 mg/kg) than in soil with 12 mg/kg. The half-life was approximately 19 days for both isomers. Only small amounts were left after one month (Van der Pas & Leistra, 1987).

The behaviour of technical grade 1,3-dichloropropene in the soil from 4 fields (soil containing 13.2-24.6% of organic matter) was studied in the laboratory. The transformation rates of *cis*- and *trans*-1,3-dichloropropene were measured in soil samples taken from the ploughed layer of the fields. Pure 1,3-dichloropropene was added at 35 µlitre/kg moist soil. The transformation in soil from one of the fields could be approximated with first-order kinetics during the whole incubation period of 21 days. The half-lives of the *cis*- and *trans*-isomers at 10 °C were 17 and 20 days, respectively. In soil from the 3 other fields, transformation of 1,3-dichloropropene with approximate first-order kinetics in the initial period of 7-14 days was followed by a period of accelerated transformation. The concentration dropped below the limit of determination (0.1 mg/kg dry soil), 14-21 days after the start of the incubation. Presumably, soil microorganisms adapted their enzymes, resulting in an increased rate of transformation (Van den Berg & Leistra, 1989).

In 6 loamy soils, transformation was gradual and pseudo first-order for 3-6 days, and then, very rapid. There was no difference between the transformation of the *cis*- and *trans*-isomers of 1,3-dichloropropene in these soils. When the initial content in dry soil was 62-80 mg/kg, less than 0.2% remained after a week (temperature 15 °C). The greatly accelerated transformation that occurred after a short time lag suggests that the soils contained microorganisms that could transform 1,3-dichloropropene effectively (Smelt et al., 1989).

Rapid transformation was found in 6 loamy soils from fields fumigated once or twice previously, as well as from fields never treated; after 7 days, less than 0.2% of the applied dose (3.7, 18, or 92 mg 1,3-dichloropropene/kg) remained. The incubation temperature was 15 °C. However, with an initial content of 470 mg/kg, the transformation was suppressed with a half-life of 33 days. In another loamy soil, which showed no accelerated transformation pattern, the pseudo half-lives increased from 4.3 to 36 days, when initial content of 1,3-dichloropropene was raised from 3.7 to 470 mg/kg (Smelt et al., 1989).

4.1.3.2 Volatilization

Volatilization and diffusion in the vapour phase are the most significant mechanisms for the environmental dispersal and dilution of 1,3-dichloropropene and 1,2-dichloropropane. Volatilization rates from soil surfaces depend on water solubility and vapour density as well as on soil properties, such as temperature and moisture content, the depth of application, and surface wind velocity. Estimates of volatilization of *cis*-1,3-dichloropropene from soil have ranged from 20 to 75%.

D-D 92 was applied to sandy clay loam soil in a polyethylene tunnel and the air in the tunnel was monitored continuously for 1,3-dichloropropene for 4 weeks. The temperature in the tunnel was 18-29 °C. D-D 92 was injected by hand at a dose rate of 225 kg/ha, at a depth of 15 cm. About 45% of the applied D-D 92 was volatilized as 1,3-dichloropropene in the first week, increasing to 54% after 4 weeks. No more than 5% was found as 1,3-dichloropropene or 3-chloroallyl alcohol in the soil at the end of the 4-week period (Sherren & Woodbridge, 1987c).

4.1.3.3 Uptake in crops

Residues in edible crops arising from the use of "MIX D/D" or 1,3-dichloropropene have only been detected in small amounts (< 0.02 mg/kg). The most obvious reason for this is the fact that crops are not normally planted until most of the product has been eliminated. Under certain conditions, where low concentrations of 1,3-dichloropropene persist for long periods of time, plants will absorb measurable quantities. Uptake has been shown to occur in potato tubers in sandy loam soil treated with ^{14}C-1,2-dichloropropane and ^{14}C-1,3-dichloropropene 6 months prior to planting (application rate 290 litre/ha). The total radioactivity (expressed as 1,3-dichloropropene equivalents) in the tubers was 7 μg/kg (Roberts & Stoydin, 1976).

Tomatoes, bush beans, and carrots absorbed ^{14}C-1,3-dichloropropene from vermiculite culture solution and sand. During 24 h, the compound was absorbed and translocated through the plants. 3-Chloroallyl alcohol was also readily absorbed, but to a lesser extent than dichloropropene. Comparison of the metabolism of 1,3-dichloropropene and 3-chloroallyl alcohol showed rapid reversion to the general carbon pool, the half-lives for 1,3-dichloropropene and 3-chloroallyl alcohol being 1.5 and 4.4 h, respectively (Berry et al., 1980).

4.1.3.4 Movement in soil

Vapour diffusion is usually the most important mode of downward movement for "MIX D/D". McKenry & Thomason (1974) injected either Telone or "MIX D/D" into a series of soils at 11 different sites in California. The moisture levels, temperatures, cultivation, and soil profiles at the sites varied. The movement was studied during 13 and 69 days. The application rates ranged from 600 up to 2300 kg/ha. It was concluded that:

- There was a substantial and downward movement of all the components.

- Downward movement was greatest in open-textured soils that were sufficiently moist but not saturated; the fumigant was detectable at a depth of a few metres.

- Downward movement was encouraged by deep cultivation in soils with horizons of low porosity.

In the United Kingdom, however, Wallace (1979) found only traces of fumigant in the 40-60 cm layer, after an injection at a depth of 18 cm. Wallace (1976a) had found comparable results in soil in Germany. In the European studies, the diffusion was slower, because the applications were made in late autumn; soils were wetter, colder, and heavier in texture. Thus, results from studies carried out under different agronomic and climatic conditions are not necessarily comparable.

The vertical and horizontal movements of 1,3-dichloropropene were studied in a tree-nursery region in the north of the Federal Republic of Germany. Sounding pipes were used to collect water samples down to a depth of 4 m using the percussion-boring method. Further borings were set to a depth of 3 m on days 10-91 after application of a formulation containing *cis-* and *trans-*1,3-dichloropropene, methylisothiocyanate and 1,2-dichloropropane at 50 ml/m^2. Soil cores were analysed. 1,3-Dichloropropene showed a rather high mobility in the soil, as it could be detected at a depth of 4 m in all soil layers on the fourth day of application. In samples of the near-surface groundwater, collected 140 days after application, a concentration of 1.36 µg 1,3-dichloropropene per litre was found. Ten to 25 m from the treated area, 1,3-dichloropropene was also found in groundwater after 59 and 140 days (Rexilius & Schmidt, 1982).

4.1.3.5 Loss under field conditions

Williams (1968) studied the loss of 1,3-dichloropropene under field conditions in sandy loam and peat soils in Canada. The application rates were approximately 1000 and 2000 litre "Mix D/D"/ha, respectively. Eight months later, samples were collected and residues determined (Table 4).

In studies in the Federal Republic of Germany, Netherlands, and the United Kingdom, only very low residues (1%) of the amount originally applied remained after 3 months in the soil (Wallace, 1976a,b; Wallace, 1979).

A comparative trial was carried out in the United Kingdom in which "MIX D/D" and 1,3-dichloropropene were injected, at a depth of 15 cm, in clay loam at concentrations of 410 and 240 litre/ha, respectively (Table 5, see also section 4.3.2 of "MIX D/D"). Samples of soil were taken at depths of 0-20 cm, 20-40 cm, and 40-60 cm, at 6 intervals up to 9½ months after application. As part of normal recommended agricultural practice,

Table 4. Recovery of cis- and trans-1,3-dichloropropene from sandy loam or peat soils, 8 months after application of 1000 or 2000 litre "MIX D/D"/ha, respectively

Soil	Depth in cm	Residue in mg/kg soil	
		cis-1,3-dichloropropene	trans-1,3-dichloropropene
Peat	0-10	1.4	3.2
	10-20	1.8	4.8
Sandy loam	0-10	-	-
	10-20	0.3	0.4

From: Williams (1968)

the soil was ploughed 5 weeks after treatment. Soil samples were analysed for residues of cis- and trans-1,3-dichloropropene, 1,2-dichloropropane, and cis- and trans-3-chloroallyl alcohol. There was no significant difference between the residues of the 1,3-dichloropropene or the 3-chloroallyl alcohol resulting from the 2 treatments. As expected, no 1,2-dichloropropane residues were detected in soil samples treated with 1,3-dichloropropene. Residues of the cis- and trans-1,3-dichloropropenes and cis- and trans-3-chloroallyl alcohols were detected in all samples up to $9\frac{1}{4}$ months after treatment and down to the 20-40 cm soil layer. Before the soil was ploughed, the concentrations of these substances showed little change, and they were present in all 3 layers, but, after ploughing, the concentrations decreased gradually (Wallace, 1979).

1,3-Dichloropropene (D-D 95 and Telone II, containing > 92%), at concentrations of 240, 280, and 290 litre/ha, was injected into the soil of 3 bulb fields in the Netherlands in the summer. Nine points were sampled per field and the samples were taken at various times down to a depth of 3 m. Within a month, the concentrations decreased to less than 0.2 mg/kg and continued to decline gradually with time (Van der Pas & Leistra, 1987).

In 2 fields in the Netherlands (soil containing 15.7-24.6% of organic matter), the spread of the fumigant (application rate 150 litre/ha) through the soil was measured. Only low fumigant concentrations (about 0.1-0.4 mg/kg) were measured at a depth of 0.3 m. Around the depth of injection (0.15-0.2 m), the ratio of

Table 5. Residues from the plot treated with 1,3-dichloropropene at 240 litre/ha[a]

Interval since application (days)	Soil depth (cm)	Concentration in soil (mg/kg)				
		1,3-dichloro-propenes		1,2-dichloro-propane	3-chloroallyl alcohol	
		cis-isomer	trans-isomer		cis-isomer	trans-isomer
3	0-20	2.02	2.54	< 0.1	1.01	1.01
	20-40	5.98	7.32	0.2	3.16	3.34
	40-60	0.14	0.15	< 0.1	1.57[b]	1.88[b]
10	0-20	6.29	7.66	0.1	1.23	1.23
	20-40	1.79	2.10	< 0.1	1.09	1.14
	40-60	0.52	0.55	< 0.1	3.01[b]	3.24[b]
23	0-20	6.10	6.10	0.2	2.39	2.39
	20-40	3.26	3.20	0.2	1.32	1.32
	40-60	0.09	0.08	< 0.1	0.04	0.04
34		NORMAL CULTIVATION (ploughing of the soil)				
40	0-20	0.95	1.10	< 0.1	0.45	0.45
	20-40	0.97	0.90	< 0.1	0.62	0.62
	40-60	0.06	0.04	< 0.1	< 0.02	< 0.02
67	0-20	0.28	0.36	< 0.1	0.70	0.70
	20-40	0.04	0.05	< 0.1	0.32	0.26
	40-60	0.11	0.09	< 0.1	0.05	0.04
At harvest 9½ months	0-20	0.08	0.06	< 0.1	0.20	0.20
	20-40	0.02[c]	0.02[c]	< 0.1	0.04	0.03
	40-60	< 0.01	< 0.01	< 0.1	< 0.02	< 0.02
Pre-treatment	0-20	< 0.01	< 0.01	< 0.1	< 0.02	< 0.02
	20-40	< 0.01	< 0.01	< 0.1	< 0.02	< 0.02
	40-60	< 0.01	< 0.01	< 0.1	< 0.02	< 0.02

[a] From: Wallace (1979).
Note: All residues are on a dry weight basis.
[b] Anomalous results.
[c] Results confirmed by GC/MS.

cis- and *trans-*isomers changed with time in favour of the *trans-*isomer. Cumulative emissions into the air over a period of 3 weeks were calculated to range from 10 to 20% of the dosage of the *cis-*isomer, and 4 to 15% of the *trans-*isomer (Van den Berg & Leistra, 1989).

4.1.3.6 Results of supervised field trials

A field study was undertaken in France in 1988, in which D-D 92 was applied to the soil prior to planting vines, and the air in the vicinity of the treated area was monitored for 1,3-dichloropropene. D-D 92 was applied at approximately 600 kg/ha at a depth of 30-40 cm. The air levels were monitored for 10 days. No samples contained 1,2-dichloropropane at levels above the limit of determination of 0.02 mg/m^3. The highest 1,3-dichloropropene concentration found during the first 24 h (perimeter of the field) was 2.1 mg/m^3 and this declined to 0.02-0.04 mg/m^3 after 10 days. Air concentrations also decreased with increasing distance, downwind (Sherren, 1990).

4.2 Bioconcentration

No data are available on bioconcentration.

4.3 Abiotic degradation

4.3.1 Photodegradation

Li (1979) obtained results comparable with those of Tuazon et al. (1984) working with ozone, by irradiation of vapour of *cis-* and *trans-*1,3-dichloropropene with a GE-RS sunlamp (see section 4.1.1). The main reaction product was 3-chloropropionyl chloride with smaller quantities of 3-chloropropionic acid, CO_2, and phosgene. In this process, the initial reaction was epoxidation of the double bond. There is evidence of the importance of a surface reaction in the atmosphere, adsorption on to particulate matter seems to be necessary for an appreciable direct phototransformation to occur. Vapour phase photolysis of 1,3-dichloropropene was not detected after prolonged simulated sunlight irradiation in a reaction chamber. Photolysis occurred on the photoreactor surface walls suggesting surface-catalysing reactions. The reaction products suggest that 12-13% was totally degraded to CO_2 after 5 days of irradiation. Over 20% was transformed to phosgene.

No data on the photolytic decomposition of the chloropropenes in water are available. Nevertheless, UVR of these chemicals in methanol, in a frozen state, or as inclusion in adamantine matrices, may cause the production of allyl radicals, by cleavage of the allylic C-Cl bond (Krijgsheld & van der Gen, 1986).

4.4 Biodegradation and biotransformation

Several studies have been performed on the persistence of 1,3-DCP in soil, after application as a fumigant. Biodegradation by soil microorganisms does occur, depending on soil type, temperature, and moisture content. The rate of disappearance ranges from a half-life of 3 days to one of 37 days, without any consistent correlation with organic matter content of the soil, or with pH. In sterile soils, the effect of temperature was minimal (Van Dijk, 1974; Tabak et al., 1981; California State Water Resources Control Board, 1983). In general, the rates of disappearance of the *cis*- and *trans*-isomers are similar and tend to increase with moisture content and temperature, conditions that may increase, not only biodegradation, but also loss by volatilization or chemical hydrolysis. Although between 15 and 80% decomposition of field applications of 1,3-dichloropropene has been shown, the large amount that can be absorbed (80-90%) can result in soil residues existing months after application is completed (Van Dijk, 1974; Roberts & Stoydin, 1976; Sittig, 1980; Krijgsheld & van der Gen, 1986).

In biodegradability studies using a synthetic medium that contained 5 mg of yeast extract/litre and was inoculated with waste water, loss of 1,3-dichloropropene was determined after 7 days of incubation. Significant degradation was observed at 5 and 10 mg of 1,3-dichloropropene/litre and gradual adaptation was shown in subcultures. The original culture degraded about 50% of the 1,3-dichloropropene in 7 days, while the third subculture was able to degrade approximately 85% at both substrate concentrations, in the same period of time (Tabak et al., 1981).

Battersby (1990a) determined the "ready biodegradability" of *trans*-1,3-dichloropropene (95.4% *trans*- and 0.3% *cis*-isomer) using the closed bottle procedure. The substance was not degraded in this system with a negligible proportion of the theoretical oxygen demand being consumed during the 28-day incubation period.

The EEC-activated sludge respiration inhibition test was used to determine the effect of a *cis*- (51.2-52.2%) + *trans*- (43.9-44.1%) mixture of 1,3-dichloropropene containing 0.33% of 1,2-dichloropropane on the respiration rate of activated sludge. The EC_{50} for this mixture was 188 mg/litre (Battersby, 1990b).

The EEC-activated sludge respiration inhibition test was also used to determine the effect of *cis*-1,3-dichloropropene (94.5-97.5% *cis*-, 1.5% *trans*-isomer and 0.25% 1,2-dichloropropane) on the respiration rate of activated sludge. The EC_{50} for the *cis*-1,3-dichloropropene was 279 mg/litre (Battersby, 1990c).

Biodehalogenation by soil organisms has been demonstrated for 1,3-dichloropropene. The fumigant appeared to be chemically hydrolysed to 3-chloroallyl alcohol and then converted to 3-chloroacrylic acid. The chlorine is removed and the intermediate products are converted to carbon dioxide and water. The rate of disappearance of 1,3-dichloropropene at 15-20 °C was 2-3.5% per day in sandy soil and up to 25% per day in clay soils. The chloroallyl alcohol disappeared at rates of 20-60% per day at 15 °C (Van Dijk, 1974). Leistra et al. (1991) incubated 1,3-dichloropropene and its transformation product 3-chloroallyl alcohol in water-saturated subsoil material at 10 °C. The times for 50% and 95% transformation ranged from 15 to 47 days and from 27 to 79 days, respectively, for 1,3-dichloropropene. The corresponding 50% and 95% transformation times for 3 chloroallyl alcohol were 0.8-4.2 and 4.0-6.5 days, respectively.

Chemical hydrolysis is the first step in the transformation of 1,3-dichloropropene. Further transformation is thought to result from microbial action; 3-chloroacrolein and 3-chloroacrylic acid have been isolated from the metabolism of 3-chloroallyl alcohol by *Pseudomonas* species (see Fig. 4) (Belser & Castro, 1971; Roberts & Stoydin, 1976).

Soil culture studies using media enriched with 1,3-dichloropropenes, 1,2-dichloropropane, and "Mix D/D" at concentrations of up to 100 mg/kg, produced abundant growth of all microorganisms tested, indicating the use of the fumigants as carbon sources. Several of these organisms (*Rhizobium leguminosarum, Bacillus subtilis, Arthrobacter globiformis*, and *Pseudomonas fluorescens*) produced greater amounts of amino acids (Altman & Lawlor, 1966; Altman, 1969). The *cis*- and *trans*-isomers of 1,3-dichloropropene have undergone biodehalogenation by a *Pseudomonas* sp. isolated from the soil.

Cis- and *trans*-1,3-dichloropropene can be chemically hydrolysed in moist soils to the corresponding 3-chloroallyl alcohols, which can be metabolized to carbon dioxide and water by *Pseudomonas* sp. (Fig. 4).

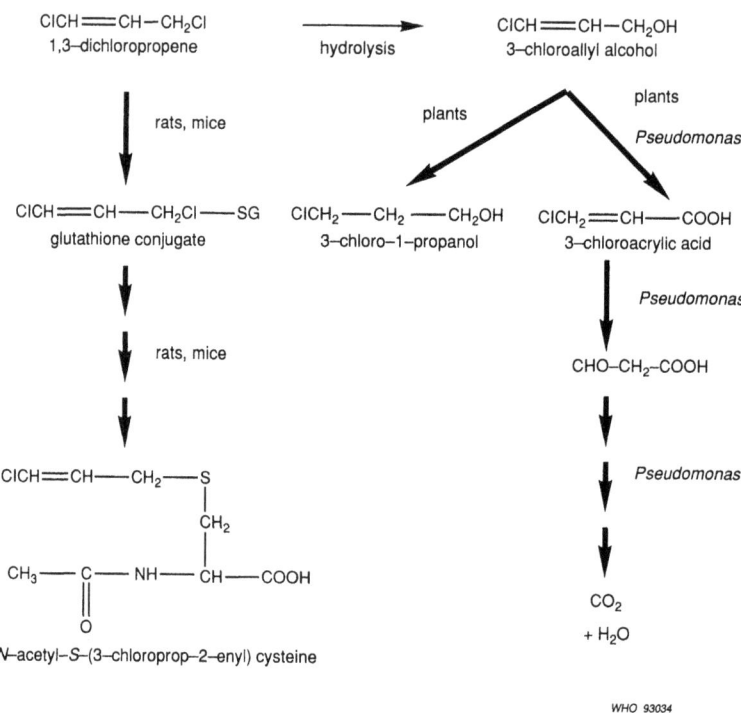

Fig. 4. Biotransformation of 1,3-dichloropropene by rodents, plants, and bacteria. Adapted from: Castro & Belser (1966); Belser & Castro (1971); Climie et al. (1979); Berry et al. (1980); and Dietz et al. (1984a,b).

The degradation of Telone II (92% 1,3-dichloropropene *cis*- and *trans*-isomers; 2% 1,2-dichloropropane and 5% mixture of propenes and hexenes, and 1% epichlorohydrin) in soil was studied using ^{14}C-1,3-dichloropropene in Fuquay loamy sand samples collected from a field in Florida. The samples were collected before, and one, and two weeks, and 2 years following application at a rate of 15 kg/ha, at depths of 0-36 cm or 36-65 cm. After 28 days incubation of ^{14}C-1,3-dichloropropene in the soil, it was degraded into $^{14}CO_2$ (44%), water-soluble metabolites (probably 3-chloroallyl alcohol), bound residues, and possibly some microbial mass. Little or no difference was observed in the degradation of ^{14}C-1,3-dichloropropene in soil samples collected one week prior to the field application of Telone II, or two weeks and two years after application. A mixed bacteria culture isolated from the soil in the presence of a carbon source, completely degraded ^{14}C-1,3-dichloropropene into $^{14}CO_2$, water-soluble products and microbial mass (Ou, 1989).

4.4.1 Miscellaneous

Laboratory experiments were conducted to determine the effects of 1,3-dichloropropene on the activity of invertase in a sandy soil. The rates of application were 30 and 60 mg/kg. No inhibition was found. The same dose levels were used to test the influence of the compound on amylase in sandy soil. After 3 days, stimulation of the formation of glucose from the added starch was seen, especially at the lowest dose level. Microbial respiration was also tested in sandy loam. The treatment did not significantly decrease oxygen consumption (Tu, 1988).

5. ENVIRONMENTAL LEVELS AND HUMAN EXPOSURE

5.1 Air

Telone II, at a rate of 293 litre/ha, was applied, at a depth of 0.45 m, simultaneously with pineapple crown planting. Each row of pineapple was covered with black polyethylene film at the time of planting. Air samples were taken inside the cover and at ground level, 10, 20, 22, 27, and 30 days after fumigation. The concentration inside the cover remained steady, at least until day 9; thereafter, a decrease was noticed and, after 22 days, the substance was no longer detectable. At ground level, the concentration fell gradually and was non-detectable after 30 days (Albrecht & Chenchin, 1985).

A small-scale, field study was undertaken in 1986, when air concentrations of 1,3-dichloropropene were measured in the vicinity of ground treated with D-D 92 (93.8%), by hand injector at a dose rate of 330 kg/ha. The air was monitored for 2 weeks. The concentration of 1,3-dichloropropene varied between 0.004 and 0.88 mg/m^3 during the first week. Levels of 1,3-dichloropropene in the second week were below the limit of determination (0.002 mg/m^3) (Sherren & Woodbridge, 1987a).

5.2 Water

An investigation of 1,3-dichloropropene in well-water in California was carried out by Maddy et al. (1982). Fifty-four wells were selected in locations of high nematocide use. No samples showed levels above the limit of determination of 0.1 µg/litre. In a survey, 72 water samples from wells in California were analysed for 1,3-dichloropropene, but no samples contained levels above 1 µg/litre (limit of determination) (Peoples et al., 1980).

Connors et al. (1990) analysed potable water samples collected in 8 homes in 3 communities in Connecticut and did not find 1,3-dichloropropene (< 0.1 µg/litre).

Dowty et al. (1975) conducted a survey on drinking-water in New Orleans, they found 1,3-dichloropropene, but did not give actual levels or frequency of occurrence.

No 1,3-dichloropropene (limit of determination 1 µg/litre) was found in 30 Canadian potable water facilities (Otson et al., 1982).

Apparently, chlorination of organic materials in water may lead to traces of 1,3-dichloropropene (< 1 µg/litre). Therefore, this process may be responsible for the observed presence of the substance in tap water (Otson et al., 1982; Krijgsheld & Van der Gen, 1986).

1,3-Dichloropropene has been identified in the waste water from a textile plant. A level of 2 µg *cis*-isomer/litre was measured in the influent of the waste water treatment plant, while higher concentrations of *cis*-1,3-dichloropropene (e.g., 6 µg/litre) were found in the effluent, together with the *trans*-isomer (0.9-4 µg/litre). Similarly, no 1,3-dichloropropene was detected in the influent of a municipal waste treatment plant, but, after "super-chlorination", a mean concentration of approximately 10 µg/litre could be detected in the liquid sludge (Krijgsheld & Van der Gen, 1986).

Hallberg (1989) reported studies on the presence of pesticides in groundwater in different States of the USA. 1,3-Dichloropropene was found only in Oregon, but no concentration(s) were reported.

Van Beek et al. (1988) examined 33 groundwater wells up to a depth of 50 m in the northern Netherlands for the presence of 1,3-dichloropropene. In this area, "MIX D/D" had been used on a large scale as a nematocide in potato growing since 1967. 1,2-Dichloropropane was present in the groundwater, but no 1,3-dichloropropene (> 0.1 µg/litre) was found in 45 samples from these wells.

Samples of upper groundwater (from 1-2 m below the water level) below 4 sandy soils were analysed in the Netherlands, for 2.5 years in 8 sampling rounds. 1,3-Dichloropropene was detected in the groundwater in 6/34 samples at concentrations in the range of < 0.1-80 µg/litre. These observations were made below fields with potato, maize, and bulb flower crops, all on low-humic to moderately humic sandy soils (Loch & Verdam, 1989).

Lagas et al. (1989) analysed groundwater (up to 6 m depth) in 5 areas (4 of which are described by Loch & Verdam, 1989), and found 1,3-dichloropropene levels above the limit of detection (0.1 µg/litre) in 2 out of 22 samples (range: < 0.1-0.2 µg/litre) taken from underneath potato crops and in 1 out of 8 samples (< 0.1-2.5 µg/litre) from below maize and bulb crops.

On 5 sites in a polder in the Netherlands, samples of surface water were taken monthly in 1987-88 and analysed. The area is situated next to the dunes (where groundwater is being pumped up for the preparation of drinking-water), and is extensively used for bulb-culture. The maximum concentration found for 1,3-dichloropropenes (*cis-* and *trans-*) was 2.5 µg/litre (Greve et al., 1989).

In the Netherlands and the Federal Republic of Germany, 1,3-dichloropropene was found in areas with extensive agriculture and horticulture. 1,3-Dichloropropene was found in the upper groundwater (depth 1-5 m) and the average levels ranged from 0.6 to 2530 µg/litre (maximum level 8620 µg/litre). In bores for irrigation (11-24 m depth), an average of 0.23 (< 0.02-0.89) µg/litre was found (Leistra & Boesten, 1989).

Ahlsdorf et al. (1989) determined the presence of 1,3-dichloropropene in the upper groundwater of an area used for potato growing, which was treated with this nematocide (about 140 kg/ha) in 1984. Very low levels of 1,3-dichloropropene (1-4 µg/litre) were found in soil with a high organic matter content, but concentrations of up to 8620 µg/litre were found in the groundwater of a clay podsol soil containing a high sand content, after one month.

1,3-Dichloropropene was detected in irrigation wells that were close to a piece of land that was treated with the chemical (10-25 m distance) in Schleswig Holstein (Germany). In the well water, concentrations of 1,3-dichloropropene varied between 0.06 and 0.89 µg/litre (Rexilius & Schmidt, 1982).

5.3 Crops

Residues in edible crop commodities, arising from the use of 1,3-dichloropropene or "MIX D/D", are reported to be generally below the limit of detection. The obvious reason for this, is the fact that crops are not normally planted until most of the product applied has dissipated. Another reason is that any 1,3-dichloropropene or "MIX D/D" taken up by the plant, would have to survive the whole crop cycle to be detected in the harvest commodity.

Supervised trials with "MIX D/D", with 23 crops in 8 countries showed that residues in edible crop commodities were below the limits of determination (< 0.01 mg/kg), for 1,3-dichloropropene, 1,2-dichloropropane, and 3-chloroallyl alcohol.

5.4 Occupational exposure

Albrecht (1987) carried out a survey to assess the exposure of 72 workers on a Hawaiian pineapple farm (attendants, crown unloaders, (truck) drivers, irrigation workers, supervisors, mulch coverers, and planters). Exposures were predominantly below 4.54 mg/m^3 (1 ppm). The concentrations in these workers ranged between 0.032 and 4.626 mg/m^3 (0.007-1.019 ppm).

Brouwer et al. (1991a) studied the inhalation of *cis*- and *trans*-1,3-dichloropropene in 12 commercial applicators in the Netherlands. The time-weighted average (TWA) concentrations of 1,3-dichloropropene ranged from 1.9 to 18.9 mg/m^3. Short-term exposure levels during tank-loading and repair ranged up to 30 mg/m^3. No correlation was observed between exposure and total area injected with 1,3-dichloropropene. Emission of 1,3-dichloropropene vapour from the soil or from spilled liquid dripping from the nozzles on to the soil may contribute to exposure.

An employee air-monitoring study to determine the amount of Telone II to which personnel would be exposed, removing soil core samples in the immediate area of the drilling, was carried out. The concentration in the air was between 0.0982 and 1.79 mg/m^3 on the first day, and between 0.202 and 3.056 mg/m^3 on second day. The time-weighted averages from personal monitoring on days one and two were 0.65 and 0.90 mg/m^3, respectively. The time-weighted averages from air monitoring on days one and two were 0.39 and 0.59 mg/m^3 (Fong & Maykoski, 1985).

A study on a single operator during a one-day application was carried out in the Federal Republic of Germany in 1986. Short-term inhalation exposures to 1,3-dichloropropene were observed during the filling operation (5.6-16.3 mg/m^3) and during nozzle changing (18.3 mg/m^3). The overall exposure during 11 h exceeded the recommended TWA value (Eadsforth et al., 1987).

An air monitoring study on exposure to 1,3-dichloropropene during the application of "Mix D/D" (not less than 50%) and D-D 92 (not less than 92%) was carried out at different locations near

Nimes in France in 1988. The 8-h time-weighted average (TWA) air concentrations of total 1,3-dichloropropene for the applicator on the 2 days of application were 11.3 and 13.2 mg/m^3, respectively, and for the tractor driver on the second day, 14.4 mg/m^3. Relatively high, short-term inhalation exposures of the applicator were measured during filling operations; the concentrations varied between 6.4 and 83.5 mg/m^3. These short-term exposures were found to contribute significantly to the overall time-weighted average exposures over the working period (Rocchi & van Sittert, 1989).

Albrecht & Chenchin (1985) found measurable concentrations of 1,3-dichloropropene in the range of 2.4-18.5 mg/m^3 during a 8-h shift in 8 out of 15 workers, planting pineapple crowns by hand, simultaneously with 1,3-dichloropropene (Telone II) treatment of the soil at 293 litre/ha.

6. KINETICS AND METABOLISM

6.1 Absorption, distribution, and elimination

6.1.1 Oral

6.1.1.1 Rat

Groups of 6 adult male and 6 female Carworth Farm E rats received, by stomach tube, 2.5-2.7 mg cis-1,3-dichloro-[2-^{14}C]propene or trans-1,3-dichloro-[2-^{14}C]propene in 0.5 ml arachis oil per rat, and excretion was followed. After 4 days, the animals were killed and the radioactivity measured in skin and carcasses. The excretion of radioactivity was very rapid, 80-90% was eliminated in the faeces, urine, and expired air in the first 24 h. The urine was the major route of elimination, i.e., 80.7 and 56.5% (average of males and females) of the dose for cis- and trans-1,3-dichloropropene, respectively. Only 2.6 and 2.2% of the 2 isomers, respectively, were eliminated in the faeces in 4 days, while 3.9 and 23.5%, respectively, were eliminated as $^{14}CO_2$ in 4 days in the expired air. Levels of the other volatile compounds in air were only 1-3% of the dose. Up to 1% of the dose in the skin and carcass was found. The difference in the amount of labelled CO_2 in expired air and urine indicated a difference in the kinetics of the 2 isomers (Hutson et al., 1971).

Groups of 8 adult Fischer 344 rats/sex were given non radiolabelled 1,3-dichloropropene at 5 mg/kg body weight, in corn oil, by gavage, for 14 consecutive days, prior to a single dose of 5 mg ^{14}C-1,3-dichloropropene/kg body weight (actual 4.5 mg) (uniformly labelled) (96.3%; 53.3% cis- and 43.0% trans-), administered to 5 out of the 8 rats on day 15. The remaining 3 rats/sex were sacrificed. The distribution of radioactivity found in the tissues (4-6%) of repeatedly dosed rats, 48 h after dosing, was similar to that of single dosed animals. There was no sex difference in the distribution of the radioactivity. In addition to the repeatedly dosed rats, 2 rats of each sex, which had not been previously dosed, received a single gavage dose of 5 mg ^{14}C-1,3-dichloropropene/kg body weight. The urine was the major route of elimination of the radioactivity derived from ^{14}C-1,3-dichloropropene, which ranged from 60 to 65% of the administered dose in 48 h in the rats with repeated doses and a single dose. Elimination of 1,3-dichloropropene as $^{14}CO_2$ was approximately (average) 26% of the administered radioactivity with about 4-5%

of the dose eliminated in the faeces, for all groups (Waechter & Kastl, 1988).

In another study, the fate of ^{14}C-*cis*- and ^{14}C-*trans*-1,3-dichloropropene (97%; 62% *cis* and 38% *trans*) was determined after a single oral dose of 1 or 50 mg/kg body weight to male Fischer 344 rats (3 animals per dose level). Urine, faeces, expired air, tissues, and remaining carcasses were analysed after 48 h. Urine was the major route of excretion, 51-61% of the administered dose being excreted over 48 h. In the carcass, 6% of the dose was found at the end of 48 h. On the basis of interval excretion data, half-lives for urinary excretion ranged from 5 to 6 h. Faeces and expired CO_2 accounted for roughly 18% and 6%, respectively. The tissue concentrations of ^{14}C activity were highest in the stomach wall, followed in decreasing order by kidneys, liver, bladder, skin, and fat (Dietz et al., 1984a,b, 1985).

6.1.1.2 Mouse

The fate of ^{14}C-*cis*- and ^{14}C-*trans*-1,3-dichloropropene (97%; 62% *cis* and 38% *trans*) was studied after oral dosing of male $B_6C_3F_1$ mice with 1 or 100 mg/kg body weight (3 animals/dose level). Urine, faeces, expired air, tissues, and remaining carcasses were analysed after 48 h. Urine was the major route of excretion, with 63 and 79%, respectively, of the administered doses (1 and 100 mg/kg body weight) being excreted over 48 h. Half-lives for urinary excretion ranged from 5 to 6 h. Faeces and expired CO_2 accounted for 15 and 14% of the ^{14}C-radioactivity, respectively. In the carcass, 2% was found. The tissue concentrations of ^{14}C-activity were highest in the stomach wall, followed in decreasing order by kidneys, liver, bladder, fat, and skin (Dietz et al., 1984a,b, 1985).

6.1.2 Inhalation

6.1.2.1 Rat

Stott & Kastl (1985, 1986) studied the pharmacokinetics of the uptake of vapours of technical grade 1,3-dichloropropene (49.3% *cis*- and 42.8% *trans*-isomer) and the disappearance of *cis*- and *trans*-1,3-dichloropropene from the blood in groups of 3-6 male Fischer 344 rats exposed to actual concentrations of 136, 409, 1362, and 4086 mg/m^3 for 3 h.

The uptake of 1,3-dichloropropene did not increase proportionately with increasing exposure concentration due to an exposure level-related decrease in the respiration rate and respiration min/volume of rats exposed to $\geq$ 409 mg 1,3-dichloropropene/m^3 and the saturation of metabolism of 1,3-dichloropropene in rats exposed to $\geq$ 1362 mg/m^3. Absorption of inhaled 1,3-dichloropropene occurred via the lungs, primarily in the lower respiratory tract (approximately 50% of total inhaled), with a small amount via the nasal mucosa (11-16%).

Following exposure to $\leq$ 1362 mg/m^3, both isomers were rapidly eliminated from the blood, with a half-life of 3-6 min. There was no interaction in the kinetics of both isomers. In addition, data obtained on rats exposed to 1362 mg/m^3 revealed that this rapid elimination phase was followed by a slower elimination phase having a half-life of 33-43 min. These data demonstrated that a combination of saturable metabolism and chemically-induced changes in respiration control 1,3-dichloropropene uptake and body-burden in rats. However, only decreases in respiration appear to influence vapour uptake.

Fisher & Kilgore (1988a) studied the excretion of the mercapturic acid of *cis*-dichloropropene in Sprague-Dawley rats. In a nose-only exposure system, groups of 3 rats were exposed for 1 h to Telone II (94%) at average concentrations of 0, 181.6, 485.8, 1289.4, 1806.9, or 3582.1 mg/m^3. Urine samples (24 h) were collected and analysed for the mercapturic derivative of *cis*-dichloropropene. At the lower exposure levels ($\leq$ 1289.4 mg/m^3), urinary excretion of the mercapturic acid derivative increased with exposure level. With exposure to 1806.9 or 3582.1 mg/m^3, no further increase was found, suggesting saturation of the metabolic process.

6.2 Influence on tissue levels of glutathione

6.2.1 Oral

Oral administration of 1,3-dichloropropene to rats or mice resulted in significant, dose-related reductions in the levels of non-protein sulfhydryls (NPS) (indicator of tissue glutathione concentration) in the forestomach and to a lesser extent in the glandular stomach and liver (Dietz et al., 1984b, 1985, see also section 6.4).

6.2.2 Inhalation

Shortly after inhalation exposure of rats to cis-1,3-dichloropropene, kidney and liver NPS contents were reduced in a dose-related manner, but returned to control values 18 h after exposure. Lung NPS levels were not affected (Stott & Kastl, 1986, see section 6.1.2.1; Nitschke & Lomax, 1990, see section 8.2.2.2).

Male Sprague-Dawley rats (200-250 g) were exposed through inhalation to 1,3-dichloropropene (Telone II, 94%) concentrations of 0, 9.1, 22.7, 150, 1384.7, 3504.9, 4335.7, or 7790.6 mg/m^3 to assess the relationship between 1,3-dichloropropene exposure concentration and tissue levels of reduced glutathione (GSH). Animals were exposed for 1 h in a dynamic, nose-only system. GSH contents were measured in the heart, kidneys, liver, lung, nasal mucosa, and testes, 2 h after 1,3-dichloropropene exposure. A decrease in nasal GSH, first seen at 22.7 mg/m^3, followed an exposure concentration-dependent curve. Exposure to concentrations above 150 mg/m^3 reduced the level of liver GSH. Lung GSH remained relatively constant at 75% of control concentrations up to 4335.7 mg/m^3. Significantly decreased GSH levels were observed in the heart, liver, lung, and testes at 7790.6 mg/m^3. Kidney GSH content was not significantly decreased. Unchanged 1,3-dichloropropene was not present in the blood of animals 2 h after exposure to 4335.7 mg/m^3 or less. Serum lactic dehydrogenase activity was affected only at 7790.6 mg/m^3. Lung weight, measured 2 and 6 h after exposure, did not differ from controls for any exposure level (Fisher & Kilgore, 1988b).

Four male Sprague-Dawley rats (200-250 g) were exposed to Telone II (94%) for 1 h, in a dynamic, nose-only exposure system. The actual 1,3-dichloropropene concentration was 354.1 ± 49.9, 703.7 ± 408.6, and 1834.2 ± 113.5 mg/m^3 (relative concentrations of cis- and trans-isomers were approximately 62 and 38%, respectively). The GSH conjugation of 1,3-dichloropropene (GSCP) in the blood of rats following exposure showed that there was no significant difference between the regression line expressed as either monophasic or biphasic decay at any exposure concentration. Moreover, no differences were found in the regression lines between the exposure concentrations. The elimination half-time of GSCP was approximately 17 h following exposure to 354.1, 703.7, or 1834.2 mg/m^3, and, thus, was not dose-dependent. This fits a one-compartment model (Fischer & Kilgore, 1989).

6.3 Biotransformation

6.3.1 Rat

In urine from rats and mice treated orally with ^{14}C-dichloropropene, no unchanged parent compound, but 2 major and 2 minor metabolites were found. The predominant metabolite was N-acetyl-S-(3-chloroprop-2-enyl) cysteine with its sulfoxide or sulfone. These data indicate that conjugation with glutathione is a major route of 1,3-dichloropropene metabolism in the rat (Dietz et al., 1984a,b, 1985) (see Fig. 4 and section 6.1.1).

Although the spontaneous reaction of *cis*-1,3-dichloropropene with glutathione is slow in the rat, the rapid urinary excretion is due to hepatic glutathione transferase, which catalyses its conjugation with glutathione. The transferase is present in the rat liver cytosol fraction and little microsomally mediated metabolism occurs. The *cis*-isomer is a better substrate than the *trans*-isomer for glutathione transferase. The conjugation then follows a classic mercapturic acid pathway (Boyland & Chasseaud, 1969). The conjugated product N-acetyl-S-(3-chloroprop-2-enyl) cysteine and its sulfoxide are excreted in the urine of rats and mice (Climie et al., 1979; Dietz et al., 1984b; van Sittert, 1984, 1989).

It has been shown that a minor metabolic pathway of the *cis*-1,3-dichloropropene is mono-oxygenase catalysed oxygenation, leading to the possible formation of the metabolite *cis*-1,3-dichloropropene-oxide (II in Fig. 5) (Van Sittert, 1989).

Rats administered 25-450 µg *cis*- and *trans*-1,3-dichloropropene/kg body weight, intraperitoneally, showed excretion of N-acetyl-S-(*cis*- and *trans*-3-chloroprop-2-enyl)-L-cysteine for 55% (*cis*-) and 45% (*trans*-) of the dose within 24 h (Onkenhout et al., 1986).

In the study of Waechter & Kastl (1988) (see section 6.1.1.1), in which rats were administered daily doses of 5 mg of non-labelled 1,3-dichloropropene/kg body weight followed by a single dose of 5 mg ^{14}-C (uniformly) labelled 1,3-dichloropropene, or a single dose of 5 mg/kg body weight, the major urinary metabolites were the mercapturic acid of 1,3-dichloropropene (1,3-D-MA) and its sulfoxide. The repeatedly dosed rats excreted slightly higher percentages of the dose as mercapturic acids than the single dosed rats (28.5% vs 22.7% for males and 25.5% vs 14.3% for females). The isomeric ratio of the 2,3-D-MA was approximately 80% *cis*- and 20% *trans*- for all groups.

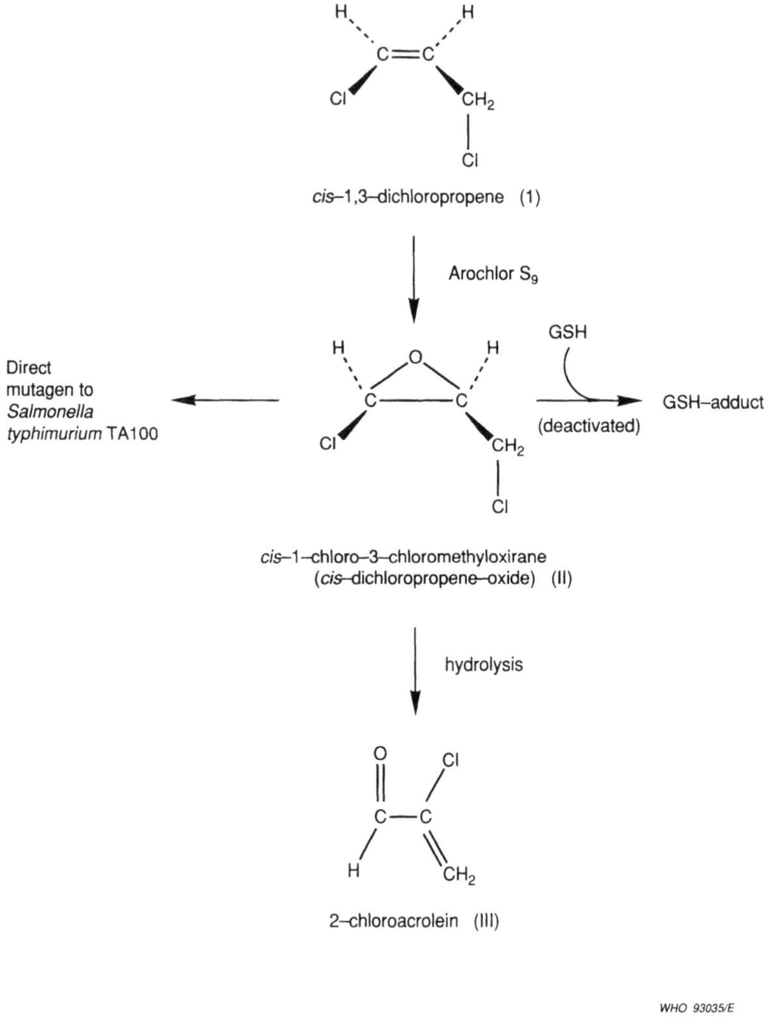

Fig. 5. Reactive mutagenic metabolites of cis-1,3-dichloropropene formed by Arochlor-induced rat liver S9 fraction (Hutson, 1984).

6.3.2 Humans

Van Welie et al. (1989, 1991) determined the relationship between respiratory occupational exposure to *cis-* and *trans-*1,3-dichloropropene and urinary excretion of 2 mercapturic acid metabolites, N-acetyl-S-(*cis-* and *trans-*)-3-chloroprop-2-enyl)-L-cysteine (*cis-* and *trans-*DCP-MA) by 12, 1,3-dichloropropene applicators in the Netherlands. Urinary excretion of these mercapturic acids followed first-order elimination kinetics. Urinary half-lives of elimination were 5.0 ± 1.2 h for the *cis-*mercapturic acid and 4.7 ± 1.3 h for the transform. These values were not statistically significantly different. A clear correlation was observed between the 8-h time-weighted average (TWA) exposure to *cis-* and *trans-*1,3-dichloropropene and complete cumulative urinary excretion of *cis-* and *trans-*DCP-MA. The *cis-*DCP-MA yielded 3 times more mercapturic acid (45%) than the *trans-* form (14%), probably because of differences in kinetics. It was concluded that the uptake of *cis-* and *trans-*1,3-dichloropropene, their metabolism to the corresponding mercapturic acids, and urinary excretion was a rapid process.

In California, applicators of 1,3-dichloropropene were also studied for personal air exposure and urinary excretion of mercapturic acid metabolites. The amount excreted was correlated with the product of the duration of exposure x TWA. The highest urinary metabolite concentration occurred during the application period, indicating rapid excretion. Skin absorption of vapour was not a significant route of exposure (Osterloh et al., 1984, 1989, see also section 9.2.1).

Air and biological monitoring of 6 operators exposed to "Mix DD" soil fumigant during filling operations in the Netherlands was carried out in 1985-86. There was rapid metabolism and elimination: the half-lives of mercapturic acid excretion were 4-5 h, with a return to background levels after 24 h. It was calculated that, under linear, non-saturation conditions, approximately 23% of the inhalation dose of the *cis-*isomer and 10% of the *trans-*isomer are excreted in the urine as mercapturic acids (Eadsforth, 1987).

6.4 Reaction with macromolecules

6.4.1 Mouse

The non-protein sulfhydryl (NPS) content, e.g., GSH, and covalent binding to macromolecules were determined in the tissues of male $B_6C_3F_1$ mice. Single oral doses of 0, 1, 5, 25, 50, or 100 mg 1,3-dichloropropene 97% (cis- 62% :trans-isomer 38%)/kg body weight were given for NPS studies and 0, 1, 50, or 100 mg ^{14}C-1,3-dichloropropene/kg body weight for binding studies. Non-glandular forestomach, glandular stomach, liver, kidneys, and bladder were analysed, 2 h after dosing. Although NPS depletion and dose-related increases in macromolecular binding were noted in several tissues of rats, these effects were more pronounced in the non-glandular stomach than in any other tissue (including glandular stomach, liver, kidneys, and bladder). The no-observed-effect level (NOEL) for NPS depletion in rat non-glandular stomach was 1 mg/kg body weight. NPS levels in non-glandular forestomach were significantly decreased at doses of 25 mg or higher and, in the liver, at 100 mg/kg body weight. Binding in the non-glandular forestomach was greatest at dose levels that caused the most depletion of tissue NPS. Limited binding occurred in the liver, kidneys, and bladder (Dietz et al., 1984b, 1985).

6.4.2 Rat

Groups of 3-9 male Fischer 344 rats (200-260 g) were administered 50 mg cis- 1,3-dichloropropene (94.1% cis- and 2.5% trans-) or 50 mg trans-1,3-dichloropropene (97.3% trans- and 0.8 cis-)/kg body weight, by gavage. The rats were sacrificed at various intervals after dosing, to determine the tissue non-protein sulfhydryls (NPS) in the liver, kidneys, forestomach, glandular stomach, and bladder. Blood samples were also taken to determine the presence of unchanged 1,3-dichloropropene. Cis-1,3-dichloropropene was only detected in the blood (6.58 µg/litre) 15 min after dosing, the blood levels of trans-1,3-dichloropropene were 11.72 and 8.38 µg/litre, respectively, 15 and 45 min after dosing. A statistically significant decrease in the non-protein sulfhydryl contents of the liver, kidneys, forestomach, and glandular stomach was found. This depletion reached a maximum, approximately 2-h after dosing. No depletion was noted in the bladder. It is not possible to distinguish the effects of cis- and trans-1,3-dichloropropene on NPS, as the results for the individual isomers were not reported. The results indicated that orally administered 1,3-dichloropropene produces a rapid and significant depletion of tissue non-protein sulfhydryls in the rat (Dietz et al., 1982).

The non-protein sulfhydryl (NPS) contents and covalent binding to macromolecules were determined in the tissues of male

Fischer 344 rats. Single, oral doses of 0, 1, 5, 25, 50, or 100 mg 1,3-dichloropropene 97% (*cis*-62% and *trans*-isomer 38%) were given for NPS studies and 0, 1, 50, or 100 mg ^{14}C-1,3-dichloropropene/kg body weight for binding studies. NPS levels in non-glandular forestomach were significantly decreased with doses of 25 mg/kg body weight or more. Binding in the non-glandular forestomach was greatest at dose levels that caused a significant depletion of tissue NPS. Limited binding was noted in the liver, kidneys, and bladder (Dietz et al., 1984b, 1985).

6.5 Appraisal

Mice, rats and humans metabolize 1,3-dichloropropene predominantly by conjugation with reduced glutathione (GSH). The glutathione conjugate is further metabolized to the corresponding mercapturic acid, which is then excreted in the urine. Consistent with the function of GSH as a detoxication mechanism, the genotoxicity of 1,3-dichloropropene was decreased in *Salmonella typhimurium* when the concentration of GSH was increased to a mammalian physiological concentration (see sections 8.6.1.2, 8.9.2).

The levels of GSH (measured as non-protein sulfhydryl content) were decreased at locations consistent with the route of exposure, i.e., predominantly in the forestomach and to a lesser extent in the glandular stomach and liver, following oral administration, and in the nasal tissue after inhalation exposure. For oral exposure, the extent of covalent binding of 1,3-dichloropropene to macromolecules was correlated with the decrease in non-protein sulfhydryl content. It is anticipated that toxic effects of 1,3-dichloropropene will occur at doses that deplete tissue sulfhydryls and will be manifested in the organs described above (forestomach, liver, and nasal tissue).

7. EFFECTS ON ORGANISMS IN THE ENVIRONMENT

The United States Environmental Protection Agency published a Health and Environmental Effects Profile for 1,3-Dichloropropene in 1985 (US EPA, 1985).

7.1 Acute toxicity

7.1.1 Microorganisms

The major effect of 1,3-dichloropropene on soil microorganisms is on nitrogen transformation. The oxidation of ammonium from soil organic nitrogen is reduced by 1,3-dichloropropene; soil ammonium levels were significantly greater and soil nitrate levels were significantly lower in soils treated with 1,3-dichloropropene compared with untreated controls (Tu, 1973; Elliot et al., 1974, 1977).

In a series of studies, the effects of 1,3-dichloropropene at 30 or 60 mg/kg soil were evaluated, in parallel, under laboratory conditions. In general, neither dose affected soil microorganisms or function appreciably. The effects of 1,3-dichloropropene on soil microorganisms and enzyme activity were not consistent in 3 soil types (sandy-, clay-, and organic soils). The numbers of fungi, 2 days after fumigation, were significantly reduced in clay and sandy soils, but not in organic soil, but recovered after 7 days. 1,3-Dichloropropene either increased or decreased the number of non-symbiotic nitrogen fixers and enzyme activity in different soils (Tu, 1978, 1979, 1981a,b).

Moje et al. (1957) studied the individual components of "MIX D/D" in old citrus soil and found that the toxicity was mainly due to its 1,3-dichloropropene content, in particular that of the *cis*-isomer (see also section 7.1.1 of "MIX D/D"). Results were as tabulated on the next page.

1,3-Dichloropropene was converted by the methanotrophic bacterium *Methylosinus trichosporium* OB3b, grown in aerobic continuous cultures. The substance was added at a concentration of 0.2 mmol/litre. After 24 h, 85% of the substance added was degraded (Oldenhuis et al., 1989).

In field experiments with continuous potato cropping, it was found that sustained annual applications of 1,3-dichloropropene

	Reduction in	
Compound	Fungi	Bacteria and actinomycetes
Cis-1,3-dichloropropene	85-95% reduction at 25 mg/kg soil	85-100% reduction at 250 mg/kg soil
Trans-1,3-dichloropropene	100% reduction at 250 mg/kg soil	100% reduction at 1000 mg/kg soil

led to insufficient control of *Globodera rostochiensis*. In the laboratory, 1,3-dichloropropene rapidly disappeared from these soils. This did not occur when the soil was sterilized. A bacterium was isolated from these soils, which was found to decompose 1,3-dichloropropene using it as a carbon and energy source. The bacterium was *Pseudomonas* sp. Repeated application of 1,3-dichloropropene led to accelerated degradation of the substance (Lebbink et al., 1989).

7.1.2 Algae

The 96-h EC_{50} value for growth, based on the concentration of chlorophyll *a* and also on cell numbers of the freshwater green algae *Selenastrum capricornutum* in a static system, was 4.95 mg/litre for 1,3-dichloropropene. The estuarine diatome, *Skeletonema costatum*, showed a 96-h EC_{50} value for growth, based on the concentration of chlorophyll *a* in culture, of 1 mg/litre (Leblanc, 1984). The EC_{50} calculated from cell numbers was 1.04 mg/litre (US EPA, 1980). The compound is moderately toxic for marine algae.

The toxicity of *cis-*, *trans-* and a mixture of *cis-* and *trans-*1,3-dichloropropenes for *Selenastrum capricornutum* was determined in a sealed 72-h growth inhibition test. The 72-h EC_{50} values (percentage reduction in area under the growth curve), expressed in terms of the mean measured concentration in the test media, were; *cis*-isomer 2.8 mg/litre; *trans*-isomer 11 mg/litre; and the mixture 8.2 mg/litre. The EC_{50} (percentage reduction in mean specific growth rate), (24-48 h) and EC_{50} (24-72 h) values determined by analysis of average specific growth rates were: *cis*-isomer 4.6 and 3.1 mg/litre; *trans*-isomer 6.6 and 7.5 mg/litre; and, for the mixture, 11 and 3.6 mg/litre, respectively (Girling, 1989a,b,c).

Rapid evaporation and sensitivity to hydrolysis are features of the chloropropenes that may interfere with proper determination of toxic concentrations of these chemicals for aquatic species, using the standard techniques. Significant loss of the test substance may have occurred during experiments carried out at temperatures above 20 °C and under "static" conditions, i.e., lasting for several days without refreshing the medium. Determination of the actual concentrations has seldom been carried out, and it is suspected that several of the data reported for the chloropropenes present an underestimation of the toxic potential of these chemicals for aquatic organisms. On the other hand, the products of hydrolysis of the chloropropenes, for instance, chloroallyl alcohols are themselves toxic (Krijgsheld & Van der Gen, 1986).

7.1.3 Invertebrates

The acute toxicity of 1,3-dichloropropene for non-target aquatic crustacea is summarized in Tables 6 and 7.

Table 6. Acute toxicity of 1,3-dichloropropene for non-target aquatic crustacea

Species	Temperature (°C)	48-h LC_{50} (mg/litre)	96-h LC_{50} (mg/litre)	Reference
Water flea (Daphnia magna)	21	0.090[a]	-	Mayer & Ellersieck (1986)
Mysid shrimp (Mysidopsis bahia)		-	0.79	US EPA (1980); Leblanc (1984)

[a] 48-h EC_{50} 6 mg/litre (US EPA, 1980; Leblanc, 1980) in a static system.

Leblanc (1980) calculated a no discernable effect concentration of 0.41 mg/litre for 1,3-dichloropropene in *Daphnia magna*, under static conditions. However, the result was based on nominal concentrations and was higher than the 48-h LC_{50} given by Mayer & Ellersieck (1986).

7.1.4 Honey bees

1,3-Dichloropropene has been tested on worker Honey bees (*Apis mellifera*) using a dusting technique. The 48-h LD_{50} was

6.6 µg/bee and 1,3-dichloropropene was rated as "relatively non-toxic" for Honey bees (Atkins et al., 1973).

Table 7. Acute toxicity of cis- and/or trans-1,3-dichloropropenes in Daphnia magna

Substance	Age	System	Temperature (°C)	48-h EC_{50} (mg/litre)	Reference
Cis-1,3 DCP (96%)	24 h	static[a]	18-22	1.4	Girling (1989a)
Trans-1,3 DCP (95.4% trans + 0.3% cis)	24 h	static[b]	18-22	3.1	Girling (1989c)
Cis- + trans- mixture (51-52% cis + 44% trans)	24 h	static[c]	18-23	3.1	Girling (1989b)

[a] pH 7.6-8.4; total hardness 176 mg/litre; dissolved oxygen 8.8-9.8 mg/litre.
[b] pH 7.8-8.1; total hardness 170 mg/litre; dissolved oxygen 8.6-9.2 mg/litre.
[c] pH 7.9-8.3; total hardness 179 mg/litre; dissolved oxygen 8.6-9.9 mg/litre.

7.1.5 Fish

The data summarized in Tables 8 and 9, suggest that 1,3-dichloropropene is moderately toxic for fish.

Heitmuller et al. (1981) exposed sheepshead minnows to 1,3-dichloropropene under static conditions. They calculated a no-observed-effect concentration of 1.2 mg/litre, but this was based on nominal concentrations.

7.1.6 Birds

Worthing & Hance (1991) reported an LC_{50} (8-day) for Mallard duck and Bobwhite quail of > 10 000 mg/kg diet.

7.2 Short-term/long-term toxicity

7.2.1 Invertebrates

No data are available.

Table 8. Acute toxicity of 1,3-dichloropropene for fish

Species	Type of test	Size (g, mm)	Temperature (°C)	96-h LC$_{50}$ (mg/litre)	References
Fathead minnow (*Pimephales promelas*)	static	0.9 g	18	4.1 (3.39-4.97)	Mayer & Ellersieck (1986)
Largemouth bass (*Micropterus salmoides*)	static	1.0 g	18	3.65[a] (3.52-3.78)	Mayer & Ellersieck (1986)
Walleye (*Stizostedion vitreum*)	static	1.3 g	18	1.08 (0.99-1.18)	Mayer & Ellersieck (1986)
Golden orfe (*Idus idus melanotus*)	-	2.8 g	20	9[b] (8-11)	Reiff (1978); Krijgsheld & Van der Gen (1986)
Sheepshead minnow (*Cyprinodon variegattus*)	static	8-15 mm	25-31	1.8[c,d] (0.7-4.5)	US EPA (1980); Heitmuller et al. (1981); Leblanc (1984)
Rainbow trout (*Salmo gairdneri*)	-	-	-	3.9	Worthing & Hance (1991)

Table 8 (contd).

Species	Type of test	Size (g, mm)	Temperature (°C)	96-h LC_{50} (mg/litre)	References
Bluegill (*Lepomis macrochirus*)	static	0.32-1.2 g	21-23	$6.1^{c,d}$ (5.1-6.8)	Buccafusco et al. (1981) US EPA (1980); Leblanc (1984)
Guppy (*Poecilia reticulata*)	semi-static	-	22	0.5^{e}	Krijgsheld & Van der Gen (1986)
Goldfish (*Carasius auratus*)	static	1.0 g	18	< 7.5	Mayer & Ellersieck (1986)

[a] Tested in hard water, 272 mg $CaCO_3$/litre.
[b] Tested in dechlorinated water, 260 mg $CaCO_3$/litre.
[c] Tested in well water, 32-48 mg/litre $CaCO_3$; pH 6.5-7.9, oxygen concentration 9.7 mg/litre reduced at the beginning to 0.3 mg/litre after 96-h exposure.
[d] Nominal concentrations.
[e] 14-day test.

Table 9. Acute toxicity of *cis*- and/or *trans*-1,3-dichloropropenes in rainbow trout (*Salmo gairdneri*)

Substance	Mean size (cm, g)	System	Temperature (°C)	96-h LC_{50} (mg/litre)	Reference
Cis-1,3 DCP (96%)	4.7 cm (1.1 g)	semi-static[a]	13-17	1.6	Girling (1989a)
Trans-1,3 DCP (95.4% *trans* + 0.3% *cis*)	4.0 cm (0.67 g)	semi-static[b]	15-17	4.5	Girling (1989c)
Cis- + *trans*- mixture (51-52% *cis* + 44% *trans*)	4.2 cm (0.68 g)	semi-static[c]	13-17	2.0	Girling (1989b)

[a] pH 7-7.8; total hardness, 226-258 mg/litre as $CaCO_3$; dissolved oxygen, 6.4-10.2 mg/litre.
[b] pH 7.2-7.8; total hardness, 234-264 mg/litre as $CaCO_3$; dissolved oxygen, 8.2-9.9 mg/litre.
[c] pH 7.5-8.3; total hardness, 251-284 mg/litre as $CaCO_3$; dissolved oxygen, 8.1-10.2 mg/litre.

7.2.2 Fish

Embryo-larval tests have been conducted on Fathead minnows (*Pimephales promelas*) exposed to 1,3-dichloropropene. The maximum no-effect concentration was 0.24 mg/litre (no details are available) (US EPA, 1980).

7.2.3 Field studies

See section 7.3.2 of "Mixtures of dichloropropenes and dichloropropane" for effects of "MIX D/D" on worms.

7.2.4 Phytotoxicity

1,3-Dichloropropene is highly phytotoxic.

8. EFFECTS ON EXPERIMENTAL ANIMALS AND *IN VITRO* TEST SYSTEMS

The United States Environmental Protection Agency, published a Health and Environmental Effects Profile for 1,3-dichloropropene in 1985 (US EPA, 1985).

In two other documents of the US EPA, health risk assessment information is given, on the basis of a comprehensive review of the toxicity data (US EPA, 1990, 1991).

8.1 Single exposures

8.1.1 Oral

The acute oral LD_{50}s for mice and rats are summarized in Table 10.

The following signs of toxicity were observed after oral administration: hunched posture, lethargy, pilo-erection, decreased respiratory rate, ptosis, diarrhoea, diuresis, ataxia, tip-toe gait, red/brown staining around the snout, tremors, emaciation, and pallor of the extremities. Haemorrhages and congestion were found in the lungs and gastrointestinal tract. The livers showed patchy areas of pallor (Jones & Collier, 1986a; Jeffrey et al., 1987; Gardner, 1989a,b,c).

8.1.2 Inhalation

The acute inhalation LC_{50}s for 1,3-dichloropropene are summarized in Table 11.

During the exposure and observation periods, the following symptoms were observed: partial closing of the eyes, pilo-erection salivation, lacrimation, lethargy, diarrhoea, reduction in respiratory rate, irregular respiratory movements (lung congestion was observed in dead animals) and hunched posture, brown staining of fur and fur loss, and reddening of ears, tail, and feet. Pathological signs were cardiopulmonary failure, acute tubular necrosis in the kidneys, and local effects on the respiratory tract.

It was suggested that the irritating properties of the vapour might serve as a warning of its presence in air. Signs of intoxication included hypoactivity, anorexia, and chromodacryorrhoea (Coombs & Carter, 1976b).

Table 10. Acute oral toxicity (LD_{50}) of 1,3-dichloropropene

Species	Concentration of substance	LD_{50} (mg/kg body weight, with 95% confidence limits)	Reference
Mouse (CD 1)	undiluted	215	Coombs & Carter (1976b)
Mouse (JCL:ICR)	92% (in corn oil)	640 (582-704)[a] 640 (547-749)[b]	Toyoshima et al. (1978a)
Rat (Fischer 344)	94.5-97.5% cis-, 1.5% trans-, 0.25% 1,2-dichloropropane, undiluted	85	Jeffrey et al. (1987); Gardner (1989b)
Rat (Fischer 344)	96.7%, trans-, undiluted	94 117[a] 78[b]	Gardner (1989c)
Rat (CD)	undiluted	127 (112-141)	Coombs & Carter (1976b)
Rat (not specified)	92% (in corn oil)	470[b] 713[a]	Torkelson & Oyen (1977)
Rat (Sprague-Dawley)	97.2%	130 (110-170)[a] between 110 and 250[b]	Jones & Collier (1986a)
Rat (Fischer 344)	D-D 95, undiluted (cis + trans 1 : 1)	57	Gardner (1989a)
Rat (Wistar)	92% (in corn oil)	560 (452-695)[a] 510 (480-726)[b]	Toyoshima et al. (1978b)
Rat (Fischer 344)	97.5%	300[a] 224[b]	Jeffrey et al. (1987)

[a] Male.
[b] Female.

A 2-h exposure to 1,3-dichloropropene at 4540 mg/m³ was lethal to rats, whereas guinea-pigs died following a single 7-h exposure to 1816 mg/m³ (Torkelson & Oyen, 1977).

One female and 3 male Rhesus monkeys (4-5 kg) were exposed to Telone II at 0, 113.5, 227, 454, 908, or 2724 mg/m³ for a single

Table 11. The acute inhalation toxicity LC_{50} for 1,3-dichloropropene (4-h exposure)

Species	Concentration of substance	LC_{50} (mg/m^3)	Reference
Rat (Wistar)	51% cis-, 43.4% trans-isomer, 1% epichlorohydrin	3309.7	Blair (1977)
Rat (Wistar)	Telone II (98.4%)	2.70-3.07[c]	Cracknell et al. (1987)
Rat (Fischer 344)	95.6% cis- and 1.5% trans-isomer	3041.8[a] 3377.8[b]	Nitschke et al. (1990)
Rat (Fischer 344)	Telone II (97.5%; 52.6% cis- and 44.9% trans-isomer)	> 3881.7-< 4698.9[a] 4014.2[b]	Streeter et al. (1987)
Rat (Crb:CD(SD)Br)	95.4% trans- and 0.3% cis-isomer	4880.5[b] 5402.6[a]	Collins (1989)

[a] male.
[b] female.
[c] mg/litre.

behavioural session of 1 h, with a 1-week recovery period after exposure. Data were obtained on all monkeys for each of the 5 atmospheric concentrations. At concentrations ranging up to 908 mg/m^3, there were no significant indications of toxicity or alterations in behaviour (the monkeys were trained to perform on a dual component FRFR (Fixed Ratio followed by a Fixed Ratio) chained schedule, with light stimulation). Only slight eye irritation was observed in all monkeys at concentrations exceeding 454 mg/m^3 (Rosenblum & Talley, 1979).

8.1.3 Dermal

The acute dermal and subcutaneous LD_{50}s are summarized in Table 12.

After dermal application, the signs of intoxication were: diarrhoea, lethargy, hunched posture, decreased respiratory rate, with lacrimation, salivation, ataxia or abasia, loss of righting reflex, diarrhoea, diuresis, and red/brown staining around the

Table 12. Acute dermal and subcutaneous LD_{50}s for 1,3-dichloropropene

Species	Route	Concentration of substance	LD_{50} (g/kg body weight, with 95% confidence limits)	Reference
Mouse (JCL:ICR)	dermal	92% (in corn oil)	> 1.211	Toyoshima et al. (1978a)
Rat (Wistar)	dermal	92% (in corn oil)	> 1.211	Toyoshima et al. (1978b)
Rat (CD)	dermal	undiluted	0.423 (0.336-0.555)	Coombs & Carter (1976b)
Rat (Sprague-Dawley)	dermal	97.2%	1.0 (0.8-1.3)[a] between 1.3 and 2.0[b]	Jones & Collier (1986b)
Rat (Fischer 344)	dermal	96.7%, trans-isomer undiluted	1.575	Gardner (1989c)
Rat (Fischer 344)	dermal	94.5-97.5% cis-, 1.5% trans-, 0.25% 1,2-dichloropropane undiluted	1.09	Gardner (1989b)
Rabbit (not specified)	dermal	92% undiluted	0.504 (0.22-1.15)	Torkelson & Oyen (1977)
Mouse (JCL:ICR)	subcutaneous	92% (in corn oil)	0.33 (0.29-0.376)[a] 0.345 (0.30-0.40)[b]	Toyoshima et al. (1978a)
Rat (Wistar)	subcutaneous	92% (in corn oil)	0.40 (0.345-0.464)[a] 0.366 (0.305-0.439)[b]	Toyoshima et al. (1978b)

[a] Male.
[b] Female.

eyes, snout or mouth. The lungs and gastrointestinal tract showed haemorrhages and irritation. Signs of skin irritation manifested by oedema, eschar formation, or subcutaneous haemorrhage were apparent (Jones & Collier, 1986b).

One 24-h application of undiluted 1,3-dichloropropene to intact, occluded New Zealand white rabbit skin caused extremely severe eschar, resulting in black necrotic tissue. The skin had hardened and was cracking after 7 days. The animals used for dermal LD_{50} estimation with 1,3-dichloropropene showed lethargy and hypothermia at dose levels above 300 mg/kg body weight (Coombs & Carter, 1976b).

8.2 Short-term exposures

8.2.1 Oral

Albino rats derived from the Wistar strain, were used in a 90-day test. Groups of 10 male and 10 female rats received doses (by gavage) of 0, 1, 3, 10, or 30 mg 1,3-dichloropropene (40% *cis*- and 28% *trans*-isomer)/kg body weight on 6 days/week. General condition, behaviour, and survival were not affected at any dose level. No distinct differences in haematological indices, serum enzyme activities, or urinalysis were observed. The relative kidney weights were significantly increased in the 30-mg group in both sexes and also in the males receiving 10 mg/kg. The relative liver weights of females at 30 mg/kg were significantly increased. Gross and microscopic examination did not reveal any abnormalities in the main organs. The 3 mg/kg body weight dose was without effect (Til et al., 1973).

8.2.2 Inhalation

8.2.2.1 Mouse

CD-1 Albino mice, 10/sex per group were exposed to production grade Telone II (whole-body exposure) at 0, 45.4, 136.2, or 408.6 mg/m^3 for 6 h/day, 5 days/week, for 90 days. No significant differences in lesions were found between the control and treated groups upon gross and histological examination, except that there were compound-related effects on the nasal turbinates. These effects were decreased height of the nasal epithelial cells resulting from a loss of cytoplasm, and disorganization of the nuclei. Necrotic cells were only observed among the females exposed to 408.6 mg/m^3. No alterations were found in the mice exposed to 136.2 mg/m^3 (Coate & Voelker, 1979a,b).

Groups of 10 male and 10 female $B_6C_3F_1$ mice were exposed (whole body) by inhalation to technical grade 1,3-dichloropropene 90.9% (*cis* 48.6% and *trans* 42.3%) containing 2.4% 1,2-dichloropropane, 5.5% mixed isomers of chlorohexane, chlorohexene, and trichloropropene, and epichlorohydrin 1.2% (as stabilizer). The actual exposures were to levels of 0, 45.4, 136, 409, or 681 mg/m^3 for 6 h/day, 5 days/week for 13 weeks. Extensive haematological, clinical-chemical, and urinalysis studies, and histopathological examination of organs and tissues were performed.

A treatment-related depression in body weight was seen at doses of 409 and 681 mg/m^3. In animals exposed to 681 mg/m^3, transient brown discoloration of the fur with a strong mercaptan odour in the coats and urine was found. The poor growth rate was reflected in a decrease or increase in the relative weights of a number of organs, but without histological alterations. An exposure-related decrease in BUN levels was observed in male mice exposed to 409 and 681 mg/m^3. Furthermore, alanine transaminase levels were increased in mice exposed to 681 mg/m^3. No other changes were found. The primary target tissues of inhaled 1,3-dichloropropenes were the nasal mucosa and urinary bladder. The changes in the nasal mucosa including slight degeneration of the olfactory epithelium and slight hyperplasia of respiratory epithelium in animals exposed to 409 and 681 mg/m^3 were dose-related. The animals also had small focal areas of nasal metaplasia, a condition in which the damaged sensory olfactory epithelium is replaced by ciliated respiratory epithelium (only in animals exposed to 681 mg/m^3).

The urinary bladders of female mice exposed to 409 and 681 mg/m^3 (7/10 and 6/10, respectively) had areas of moderate hyperplasia of the transitional epithelium (7-10 layers thick in contrast with 2-3 layers in control mice). Submucosal aggregates of lymphoid cells in the bladder, not associated with hyperplasia and not treatment-related, were found in female mice exposed to concentrations of 136 mg/m^3 or more. No treatment-related effects were found in mice exposed to 45.4 mg/m^3 (Stott et al., 1984, 1988).

8.2.2.2 Rat

Fischer 344 rats, 10/sex per group, were exposed to 0, 45.4, 136, or 409 mg/m^3 of production grade Telone II, for 6 h/day, 5 days/week for 90 days. No significant differences in lesions were found between the control and treated groups on gross or histological examination, except that compound-related effects on the nasal turbinates were found. These effects included decreased height of the nasal epithelial cells resulting from a loss of cytoplasm, and a disorganization of the nuclei. Necrotic cells were observed in all of the male and female rats exposed to 409 mg/m^3 and in 6/10 of the female rats exposed to 136 mg/m^3. No alterations were found in the animals with 45.4 mg/m^3 (Coate & Voelker, 1979a,b).

Groups of 5 male rats were exposed to atmospheres containing concentrations of 1,3 *cis-/trans*-dichloropropene (92%) of 0 or 13.6 mg/m^3 for 0.5, 1, 2, or 4 h/day, 5 days/week for 6 months. The only effect in all the exposed groups was a slight, apparently reversible change, seen microscopically in the kidneys of male rats (Torkelson & Oyen, 1977).

Groups of 24 male and 24 female rats were exposed repeatedly to air containing 0, 4.54, or 13.6 mg 1,3-dichloropropene/m^3 for 7 h/day, 5 days/week for 6 months. Changes attributable to 1,3-dichloropropene were limited to cloudy swellings in the renal tubular epithelium of male rats in the 13.6 mg/m^3 group. Female rats in this group showed an increased liver to body weight ratio, though no histopathological changes were observed. A recovery group of male and female rats was maintained for 3 months following the 6-month exposure to 4.54 or 13.6 mg/m^3. No changes were observed in the renal epithelium following this recovery period (Torkelson & Oyen, 1977).

In a well-designed study (Stott et al., 1984, 1988), groups of 10 male and 10 female Fischer 344 rats were exposed through inhalation to technical grade 1,3-dichloropropene 90.9% (for composition see section 8.2.2.1) in actual concentrations of 0, 45.4, 136, 409, or 681 mg/m^3, for 6 h/day, 5 days/week for 13 weeks. Haematological, clinical-chemical studies, urinalysis, and histopathological studies of organs and tissues were carried out.

In the rats exposed to 681 mg/m^3, transient brown discoloration of the fur with a strong mercaptan odour in the coats and urine was found. The body weights of rats exposed to 409 or 681 mg/m^3 were decreased in an exposure-related manner. The relative weights of the testes were increased and thymus weights decreased. Rats exposed to 409 and 681 mg/m^3 had slightly lower levels of serum proteins. No other treatment-related changes in clinical-chemical or haematological parameters were found.

The primary target tissues of inhaled 1,3-dichloropropenes were the nasal mucosa in male and female rats and the uteri in females. The effects consisted of dose-related degenerative effects on the nasal olfactory epithelium or mild hyperplasia of the respiratory epithelium or both, in all animals exposed to 409 and 681 mg/m^3, and 2 of the 10 male animals in the 136 mg/m^3 group.

The uteri of 7 out of 10 female rats exposed to 681 mg/m^3 were not developed as completely as those of control animals, suggesting hypoplasia of the uterine tissues. The only other change noted histologically was the atrophic appearance of the mesenteric adipose tissue in the rats exposed to 681 mg/m^3. No treatment-related effects were observed in rats of either sex exposed to 45.4 mg 1,3-dichloropropenes/m^3 (Stott et al., 1984, 1988).

In a study to investigate the effects of 1,3-dichloropropene on tissue sulfhydryl levels, groups of 15 male and 15 female Fischer 344 rats were exposed to vapours of *cis*-1,3-dichloropropene (94.3-95.6% *cis*-, 1.5% *trans*-1,3-dichloropropene and 0.2% 1,2-dichloropropane) at 0, 45.4, 272.4, or 681.0 mg/m^3 for 6 h/day, 5 days/week for 9 exposures. Whole-body exposures occurred under dynamic air-flow conditions. On the day after the last exposure, 5 males and 5 females/dose level were necropsied. Major organs were weighed and selected tissues were evaluated histopathologically. Groups of 5 animals/sex per dose level were used to determine the non-protein sulfhydryl (NPS) contents of the liver, kidneys, and lung, 1 and 18 h following the last exposure.

Rats exposed to 681 mg/m^3 lost weight, but not those exposed to 272.4 mg/m^3. There were concentration-related decreases in liver, kidney, and lung NPS levels in male rats, when measured after 1 h. After 18 h, the NPS levels were higher than those of the controls and there were no associated gross or histopathological changes in these organs. The NPS measurements for females were unremarkable. Histopathological examination revealed changes of moderate severity in the respiratory and olfactory mucosa in the nasal cavity of males and females exposed to 681 mg/m^3. There were no changes in the animals exposed to 272.4 mg/m^3 (Nitschke & Lomax, 1990).

Groups of 10 male and 10 female Fischer 344 rats (6 weeks old) were exposed to *cis*-1,3-dichloropropene at 0, 45.4, 136, or 409 mg/m^3 for 6 h/day, 5 days/week for 13 weeks. The test material was reported to consist of 94.3% (95.6%) *cis*-1,3-dichloropropene, 1.5% *trans*-1,3-dichloropropene and 0.2% 1,2-dichloropropane. Whole-body exposures occurred under dynamic conditions. No exposure-related effects were noted in haematology or clinical chemistry. At 409 mg/m^3, body weights of male rats were significantly decreased compared with controls throughout the 13-week exposure period; body weights of female rats were significantly decreased during the first 6 weeks, but were comparable with those of the controls at the end of the study. As a result of the decreased body weight in male rats, the relative liver, kidney, lung, and testes weights were significantly elevated in comparison with control values. The relative liver weight in females was also increased. These organ weight changes were not accompanied by gross or histopathological changes. Exposure-related changes only occurred in the nasal cavities of the rats of both sexes exposed to 409 mg/m^3 and consisted of multifocal bilateral degeneration of olfactory epithelium and slight bilateral multifocal hyperplasia of respiratory epithelium. No effects were noted in rats exposed to 45.4 or 136 mg/m^3. The NOEL was considered to be 136 mg *cis*-1,3-dichloropropene/m^3 (Nitschke et al., 1991).

8.2.2.3 Other animal species

Groups of 12 male and 12 female guinea-pigs, 3 male and 3 female rabbits and 2 dogs were exposed repeatedly to air containing 0, 4.54, or 13.6 mg 1,3-dichloropropene/m^3 for 7 h/day, 5 days/week for 6 months. No changes resulting from 1,3-dichloropropene exposure were observed in guinea-pigs, rabbits, or dogs (Torkelson & Oyen, 1977).

8.3 Skin and eye irritation, sensitization

8.3.1 Skin irritation

1,3-Dichloropropene is extremely irritating to the skin (Worthing & Hance, 1991).

Telone II (52.63% *cis*- and 44.91% *trans*-1,3,-dichloropropene), 0.5 ml, was applied for 4 h to the back (clipped free of fur) of 2 male and 4 female New Zealand White rabbits. After 4 h, the wrapping and gauze patch and any residual test substance were removed. Dermal irritation characterized as slight to moderate erythema and moderate to severe oedema was observed at the site of application immediately following the 4 h exposure period. Subsequent observations revealed slight to moderate erythema, oedema, and exfoliation. These changes were still present in some of the animals after 14 days (Jeffrey, 1987a).

In a 4-h rabbit skin irritancy test, undiluted *cis*-1,3-dichloropropene (94.5-97.5% *cis*-, 1.5% *trans*-1,3-dichloropropene and 0.25% 1,2-dichloropropane) caused well defined erythema and moderate oedema shortly after removal of the semi-occlusive dressings in New Zealand White rabbits (3-5 months of age). After removal of the dressings, the skin was washed after 4 h. Resolution of the irritancy reaction was first apparent on the day after treatment and was complete within 14 days (Gardner, 1989b).

In another 4-h rabbit skin irritancy test, 0.5 ml of undiluted *trans*-1,3-dichloropropene (96.7%) caused irritation not exceeding well-defined erythema and slight oedema. New Zealand White rabbits (3-5 months of age) were used. After the 4-h exposure, the dressings were removed and the skin washed. Resolution of the irritation was first apparent 72 h after treatment and was complete by day 21 (Gardner, 1989c).

8.3.2 Eye irritation

1,3-Dichloropropene is a severe eye irritant (Worthing & Hance, 1991).

Aliquots of 0.1 ml Telone II (52.63% *cis*- and 44.91% *trans*-1,3-dichloropropene) were instilled into the conjunctival sac of one eye of 4 male and 2 female New Zealand White rabbits. The eyes of all rabbits remained unwashed. Slight to marked redness and slight to moderate chemosis were found after the treatment. The treated eyes had a slight to marked amount of discharge as well as reddening of the iris. In one animal, opacity was found which resolved as did all the other changes within 14 days following treatment (Jeffrey, 1987b).

In the rabbit eye irritancy test, 0.1 ml *trans*-1,3-dichloropropene (96.7%) caused moderate to severe conjunctival irritation and minor irritation changes of the cornea (opacities), chemosis, and iridial responses within 24 h following instillation into the eye. Resolution of the irritant effects of *trans*-1,3-dichloropropene was advanced 7 days after treatment and complete one week later. There was an initial pain response (Gardner, 1989c).

Ten male and 10 female Sprague-Dawley rats (*Spartan substrain*) were exposed to an aerosol (mean size 2.96 µm; 99% of particles were 6 µm or less in diameter) in a glass chamber for 1 h at a nominal concentration of 5.2 mg/litre of air. Five male and 5 female animals were maintained under ambient conditions as controls. Slight transitory eye irritation was observed during the exposure (Yakel & Kociba, 1977).

8.3.2.1 In vitro studies

The corneal thickness of isolated eye preparations subjected to application of *cis*-1,3-dichloropropene (94.5-97.5% *cis*-, 1.5% *trans*-1,3-dichloropropene and 0.25% 1,2-dichloropropane) increased by more than 20% within 3 h. The isolated rabbit eye test described by Price & Andrews (1985) was used. Corneal uptake of fluorescein was demonstrated at the conclusion of the test. The results indicated that application of *cis*-1,3-dichloropropene to the eye *in vivo* would cause significant tissue damage (Gardner, 1989b).

8.3.3 Sensitization

1,3-Dichloropropene was applied in corn oil in a 5% v/v concentration 3 times topically to the skin of guinea-pigs followed by a 1% concentration as a challenge following the method of Buehler (1965). A positive reaction was obtained in 5 out of 20 guinea-pigs of the "P" strain. The reaction was considered to be mild to moderate skin sensitization (Coombs & Carter 1976b).

Ten male, Hartley albion guinea-pigs received 3 dermal applications on the back of 0.4 ml of 0.1% (v/v) Telone II (52.63% *cis*- and 44.91% *trans*-1,3-dichloropropene) in mineral oil; another group received only the vehicle during the induction phase of the study. The dermal sensitization potential was tested using the modified Buehler method. A positive control group received 2 applications of 10% epoxy resin and a third application of 5% epoxy resin. All groups were challenged dermally 2 weeks after the last induction application. The control group did not show any signs of sensitization, while 5 out of the 10 animals of the positive control group revealed slight erythema. Nine out of 10 guinea-pigs challenged with 0.1% Telone II revealed slight to moderate erythema. Telone II was considered a potential skin sensitizer at the concentrations tested (Jeffrey, 1987c).

In the guinea-pig maximization test of Magnusson & Kligman, all 20 test animals showed positive responses, 24 and 48 h after removal of the challenge patches. Guinea-pigs of the Dunkin-Hartley strain (5-9 weeks of age) were used in this study. In a study by Gardner (1989b), 0.1% *cis*-1,3-dichloropropene (94.5-97.5% *cis*-, 1.5% *trans*-1,3-dichloropropene and 0.25%

1,2-dichloropropane) was injected intradermally; topical induction was carried out using a 5% solution in corn oil, and the topical challenge using 2.5% in corn oil.

In the guinea-pig maximization test of Magnussen & Kligman, 16 out of 20 test animals showed positive responses 24 and/or 48 h after removal of the challenge patches. Guinea-pigs of the Dunkin-Hartley strain (age 5-9 weeks) were used. Intradermal injection, carried out at concentrations of 0.05% *trans*-1,3-dichloropropene (96.7%) or more resulted in red areas with defined edges. The concentration selected (10%) for topical induction did give slight irritation, but the concentration for the topical challenge of 5% was without effect. The solvent was corn oil (Gardner, 1989c).

8.4 Long-term exposure

See section 8.7 (Carcinogenicity).

8.5 Reproduction, embryotoxicity, and teratogenicity

8.5.1 Reproduction

8.5.1.1 Inhalation (rat)

Groups of 30 male and 30 female Fischer 344 rats (6 weeks of age) were exposed to Telone II (1,3-dichloropropene containing 2% epoxidized soybean oil) at 0, 45.4, 136, or 409 mg/m^3 (first 7 days of study: 0, 22.7, 90.8, or 272.4 mg/m^3) for 6 h/day, 5 days/week during the premating period and for 7 days/week during breeding, gestation, and lactation, for 2 generations. The Telone II used had a purity of 92% and the remainder of the test material comprised chlorinated and unchlorinated alkanes and alkenes as well as approximately 2.0% epoxidized soybean oil. Following 10 weeks of exposure, the adult rats (F_0) were mated twice to produce the F_{1a} and F_{1b} litters. After weaning, 30 pups/sex per exposure from the F_{1b} litters were selected and, after 12 weeks, used to produce the F_{2a} and F_{2b} litters.

All litters were examined on the day of parturition, the following indices of fertility being recorded: gestation length, litter size, pup survival indices, number of live pups on days 1 up to 28 postpartum, sex and weight of litters, lactation and individual body weights, and any visible physical abnormalities. Gross necropsy was carried out on adult rats F_0 and F_1 and weanling F_{1b} and F_{2b} rats and histopathological studies on adult rats. Inhalation of up to 409 mg/m³ for 2 generations did not adversely affect reproduction or neonatal growth or survival. Exposure to 409 mg/m³ resulted, however, in parental toxicity (F_0, F_1), as indicated by decreases in body weight and histopathological effects in the nasal mucosa (slight, focal hyperplasia of the respiratory mucosal epithelium and/or focal degenerative changes in the olfactory epithelium). No adverse effects were observed in the parents in the 136 mg/m³ group. The reproductive no-effect level was 409 mg/m³ (Breslin et al., 1987, 1989).

8.5.1.2 Intraperitoneal (mouse)

1,3-Dichloropropene (Telone II) in corn oil was injected intraperitoneally in $B_6C_3F_1$ male mice (4 per group) at dose levels ranging from 10 mg up to 600 mg/kg body weight, daily for 5 days, to study sperm morphology, epididymal sperm counts, and testes weights. Testicular toxicity was assessed at day 35. No animals survived at dose levels of 150 mg/kg body weight or more. No effects on the testes were found at dose levels up to 75 mg/kg body weight (Osterloh et al., 1983).

8.5.2 Teratogenicity

8.5.2.1 Inhalation (rat)

In a range-finding study, groups of 7 or 8 female Fischer 344 rats were exposed to Telone II (92.1%; 47.7% *cis*- and 42.4% *trans*-1,3-dichloropropene, impurities, and 1.8% epichlorohydrin) at 0, 230, 680, or 1360 mg/m³ for 6 h/day on days 6-15 of gestation.

Consumption of food and drinking-water was decreased during the period of exposure in rats exposed to 680 or 1360 mg/m³ and the rats showed a significant decrease in body weight gain. Rats were sacrificed on day 16 and examined. During exposure, nasal exudate and red crusty material around the eyes were observed. In the group exposed to 1360 mg/m³, a significant decrease in litter size and significant increase in resorption were seen, while in the groups exposed to 230 and 680 mg/m³, the same changes were observed, but were not statistically significant (Kloes et al., 1983).

Groups of 30 Fischer 344 rats were exposed, via inhalation, to 1,3-dichloropropene 90.1% (47.7% *cis*- and 42.4% *trans*-isomer) at 0, 91, 272, or 545 mg/m³ air for 6 h/day on days 6-15 of gestation. Food consumption and maternal body weight gain were depressed in all treated groups in a dose-related manner. A decrease in water consumption was found in rats at the highest dose-level. No consistent or dose-related effects on reproductive performance were found. The number of implantations, resorptions, litter size, fetal weights, and fetal lengths were comparable with the controls. A slight, but statistically significant, dose-related increase in the incidence of delayed ossification of the vertebral centra was found in rats, but considered of little toxicological significance in the light of the maternal toxicity observed. The authors stated that there was no evidence of a teratogenic or embryotoxic response at exposure levels up to and including 545 mg/m^3 (John et al., 1983; Hanley et al., 1987).

8.5.2.2 Inhalation (rabbit)

In a range-finding study, groups of 7 New Zealand White rabbits were exposed to Telone II (92.1%, 47.7% *cis*- and 42.4% *trans*-1,3-dichloropropene, impurities and 1.8% epichlorohydrin) at 0, 230, 680 or 1360 mg/m^3 for 6 h/day on days 6-18 of gestation. The rabbits were sacrificed on day 19 and examined. Six out of 7 rabbits exposed to 1360 mg/m^3 showed signs of toxicity, such as rear limb ataxia, decreased or absence of righting reflex, and flaccid hind limb muscles; these animals died or were sacrificed. Histologically, no effects were detected in the brains of these animals. Maternal body weight was statistically significantly decreased during exposure in the 680 mg/m^3 group, but weights in the 230 mg/m^3 group were comparable with those of the controls. There were no differences in the reproductive parameters between the groups exposed to 230 and 680 mg/m^3 and the controls. No teratological effects were found (Kloes et al., 1983).

Groups of 25-31 inseminated New Zealand white rabbits were exposed to 1,3-dichloropropene 90.1% (47.7% *cis*- and 42.4% *trans*-isomer) at 0, 91, 272, or 545 mg/m^3 air for 6 h/day on days 6-18 of gestation. Decreased weight gain was observed among rabbits at 272 and 545 mg/m^3, but no pronounced maternal toxicity was observed. No evidence of teratogenic or embryotoxic responses was observed (John et al., 1983; Hanley et al., 1987).

8.6 Mutagenicity and related end-points

8.6.1 In vitro studies

8.6.1.1 Microorganisms

Cis- and *trans-*1,3-dichloropropene or a mixture were tested for their mutagenic activity in *Salmonella typhimurium* and in *Saccharomyces cerevisiae*, with and without metabolic activation. Most of the studies showed a positive effect, especially with *Salmonella typhimurium* TA100 and TA1535, with, and without, metabolic activation. With TA98 and TA1537, positive and negative effects were found. *Saccharomyces cerevisiae* was positive. The results are summarized in Table 13. Samples of highly purified 1,3-dichloropropene or *cis-*1,3-dichloropropene, however, were not mutagenic to *Salmonella typhimurium* TA100, indicating that trace impurities, such as 1,3-dichloropropene oxide, were the cause of the activity (Talcott & King, 1984; Watson et al., 1987, see section 8.8.2).

There was a difference in mutagenicity (expressed as rev/μmol) between the *cis* and *trans* isomers of 1,3-dichloropropene in *Salmonella typhimurium* TA100, with, and without, metabolic activation. The *cis-*isomer induced a greater number of revertants, with, and without, S9 mix, than the *trans-*isomer and also showed stronger alkylating properties in the NBP-test. Furthermore, a longer preincubation time invariably led to higher mutagenic activity, and an increase in protein added to the activating system increased the efficiency of the metabolic activation (Neudecker et al., 1980, Neudecker & Henschler, 1986).

Salmonella typhimurium TA100 was used to test for the mutagenicity of *cis-* and *trans-*3-chloroallyl alcohol (99%), with, and without, metabolic activation. No mutagenicity was observed without S9 mix, over a range of 0.01-1000 μg/plate. However, a positive effect was obtained with S9 mix and *cis-*3-chloroallyl alcohol (in high concentration) (Connors et al., 1990).

Von der Hude et al. (1988) used the SOS chromotest with *Escherichia coli* PQ 37, to examine 1,3-dichloropropene (in DMSO) at concentrations of 0, 1.0, 3.3 or 10.0 mmol/litre, without S9. In this strain, the structural gene for beta-galactosidase lacZ is placed under the control of the SOS-gene sfiA. The expression of this gene, induced by DNA-damage, is measured indirectly by determination of the beta-galactosidase activity. The test was positive with concentrations of 1.0 mmol/litre or more.

Table 13. Mutagenicity tests with 1,3-dichloropropenes (1,3-DCP) on microorganisms

Substance	Organism/strain	Dose	Type of test	Metabolic activation	Result	Reference
Cis-1,3-DCP (99.9%)	Salmonella typhimurium TA1535, TA1537, TA1538	0.1-1.0 µg/ml	top agar	S9 mix/none	+	Neudecker et al. (1977) Kier et al. (1986)
Cis-1,3-DCP (> 99%)	TA98, TA100, TA1535	20-2000 µg	plate	S9 mix/none	+	Brooks et al. (1978)
	TA1538	20-2000 µg	plate	S9 mix/none	-	Brooks et al. (1978)
Cis-1,3-DCP (96.3% + trans-1,3-DCP 1.5%, + 1,2-DCP 0.25%)	TA100, TA1535	78-1250 µg/ml	*	S9 mix/none	+	Brooks & Wiggins (1990)
	TA98, TA1537, TA1538	78-1250 µg/ml	*	S9 mix/none	-	Brooks & Wiggins (1990)
Cis-1,3-DCP	TA100, TA1535, TA1978	20-100 µg	plate	S9 mix/none	+	DeLorenzo et al. (1977) Kier et al. (1986)
Trans-1,3-DCP (97.5%)	TA1535, TA1537, TA1538	0.1-1.0 µg/ml	top agar	S9 mix/none	+	Neudecker et al. (1977) Kier et al. (1986)
Trans-1,3-DCP	TA100, TA1535, TA1978	20-100 µg	plate	S9 mix/none	+	DeLorenzo et al. (1977) Kier et al. (1986)

Table 13 (contd).

Trans-1,3-DCP (98% + cis-1,3-DCP 0.3%)	TA100, TA1535	39-1250 µg/ml	*	S9 mix/none	+	Brooks & Wiggins (1989a)
	TA98, TA1537, TA1538	39-1250 µg/ml	*	S9 mix/none	-	Brooks & Wiggins (1989a)
1,3-DCP (51.3% cis, 43.7% trans, 0.6% epichlorohydrin)	TA100, TA1535	20-2000 µg	plate	S9 mix/none	+	Brooks et al. (1978)
	TA98, TA1538	20-2000 µg	plate	S9 mix/none	±	Brooks et al. (1978)
1,3-DCP ***	TA100, TA1535	3-333 µg/ml	plate	S9 mix/none	+	Haworth et al. (1983)
	TA98, TA1537	3-333 µg/ml	plate	S9 mix/none	-	Haworth et al. (1983)
1,3-DCP ***	TA100, TA1535	1000 µg/ml	*	S9 mix/none	+	Priston et al. (1983)
	TA98, TA1537	1000 µg/ml	*	S9 mix/none	-	Priston et al. (1983)
1,3-DCP ***	TA100	0.1-10 µmol	plate	S9 mix/none	+	Stolzenberg & Hine (1980)
1,3-DCP ***	TA98	100 µg	**	none	+	Vithayathil et al. (1983)

Table 13 (contd).

Substance	Organism/strain	Dose	Type of test	Metabolic activation	Result	Reference
1,3-DCP ***	*Saccharomyces cerevisiae* JD1	1000 or 5000 µg/ml	liquid suspension culture	S9 mix/none	+	Priston et al. (1983)
Cis-1,3-DCP (96.3% + trans-1,3-DCP 1.5% + 1,2-DCP 0.25%)	*Escherichia coli* WP2 UVRA pKM 101	78-1250 µg/ml	*	S9 mix/none	+	Brooks & Wiggins (1990)
Trans-1,3-DCP (98% + cis-1,3-DCP 0.3%)	WP2 UVRA pKM 101	39-1250 µg/ml	*	none S9 mix	- +	Brooks & Wiggins (1989a)

* Assays were performed by the pre-incubation method in sealed containers.
** Salmonella/microsome multiple indicator test.
*** Details of composition not given.

8.6.1.2 Effects of glutathione on bacterial mutagenesis

The addition of glutathione (GSH), at physiological concentrations, to *in vitro* bacterial test systems of *Salmonella typhimurium* TA100 has shown a clear protective effect, i.e., a virtual elimination of the mutagenic response of 1,3-dichloropropene (Brooks et al., 1978; Climie et al., 1979; Creedy & Hutson, 1982; Wright & Creedy, 1982; Creedy, 1983; Creedy et al., 1984; Brooks & Wiggins, 1990). This protective effect occurs in either the presence or the absence of S9 for both the (*cis*)- and (*trans*)-isomers. Protection, in the presence of S9, is consistent with the operation of glutathione transferase enzyme occurring in the added S9 fraction. This enzyme is also present in mammalian cells, and as the metabolic studies have shown, it plays a key role in the rapid detoxification of *cis*-1,3-dichloropropene in mammalian tissue (Climie et al., 1979; Brooks & Wiggins, 1991).

Even in the absence of S9, this protection by GSH still exists against the mutagenic action of 1,3-dichloropropene. Thus, it is likely that an additional mechanism for protection exists that probably reflects a reaction between the mutagenic component(s) and GSH. This additional mechanism may also play an important role in the detoxification of 1,3-dichloropropene via a spontaneous nucleophilic substitution reaction between the chloromethyl carbon of 1,3-dichloropropene and the sulfur atom of glutathione.

These 2 mechanisms with GSH afford complete protection against the mutagenic activity of the *trans*-isomer in bacterial test systems, in the presence and absence of S9 (Hutson & Stoydin, 1977; Creedy & Hutson, 1982; Wright & Creedy, 1982).

In the presence of Aroclor-induced rat liver S-9 fraction and a rat liver microsomal mono-oxygenase system, *cis*-1,3-dichloropropene (I) is apparently metabolized to a mutagenic metabolite, *cis*-1-chloro-3-chloromethyloxirane (II), which is not as effectively deactivated by glutathione as the parent compound. *Cis*-dichloropropeneoxide was shown not to be stable in aqueous medium, 2-chloroacroleine (III) was the product of hydrolysis, another direct-acting mutagen for *Salmonella typhimurium* TA100 (Hutson, 1984) (see Fig. 5). Glutathione transferase systems afford efficient protection against this bioactivated product of 1,3-dichloropropene. The protective action of glutathione-linked systems against the mutagenicity observed in *S. typhimurium* has also been shown to occur *in vivo*.

8.6.1.3 Mammalian cells

In a gene mutation assay, V79 Chinese hamster cells were exposed to *cis*-1,3-dichloropropene (99.9%) in DMSO at dose levels of 2.5 to 20 µg/ml. No indication for an increased mutation frequency at the HGPRT locus was found in these cells (Meyer, 1980).

Telone II (48.9% *cis*- and 43.2% *trans*-1,3-dichloropropene) was tested in the Chinese hamster ovary cell/HGPRT mutagenicity assay, with the cell line designated as CHO-K1-BH4, with, and without, metabolic activation. Three tests were carried out without activation. The first test with 50, 100, 150, 200, and 250 mmol/litre, showed an increase in mutation frequency at the 200 and 250 mmol/litre dose levels. However, the biological significance is doubtful because of the extreme toxicity at these high dose levels. In a repeat of this study using the same concentrations, no increase in mutation frequency was found. The results of a third study using concentrations of 50, 100, 125, 150, and 200 mmol/litre were also negative. The fourth test was with activation, with dose levels of 50, 100, 125, 150, and 200 mmol/litre. The relative survival ranged from 98% at 50 mmol/litre to 14% at 200 mmol/litre. No increase in mutation frequency was observed. The results indicated that Telone II was not mutagenic in the CHO/HGPRT assay, with, or without, metabolic activation (Mendrala, 1986).

8.6.1.4 DNA damage

Cis- and *trans*-1,3-dichloropropene were tested for their ability to induce unscheduled DNA synthesis (UDS) in Hela S_3 cells. The lowest dose, 10^{-4} mol/litre was the dose at which UDS occurred, the dose-response curves being rather shallow (Schiffmann et al., 1983).

Telone II (49.5% *cis*- and 42.6% *trans*-1,3-dichloropropene) was evaluated in the rat hepatocyte unscheduled DNA synthesis assay at concentrations from 1×10^{-6} up to 3×10^{-3} mol/litre. In an initial and a repeat assay, toxic effects on the hepatocyte cultures (indicated as detachment of the cells and/or a granular appearance) occurred at 1×10^{-5} mol/litre and at 1×10^{-4} mol/litre or more, respectively. In both tests, Telone II failed to elicit significant DNA repair in the primary cultures of rat hepatocytes, over the wide range of concentrations tested, suggesting an apparent lack of genetic activity (Mendrala, 1985).

The liquid *Bacillus subtilis* strain H17 (arg-, trp-, recE+) microsome rec-assay was used to evaluate the DNA-damaging effect of 1,3-dichloropropene with, and without, S9 mix. The concentrations of 1,3-dichloropropene used with, and without, S9 mix were for CR50Rec+/CR50Rec-, 7.62 x 10 / 2.49 x 10 and 4.79 x 10^2/1.01 x 10^3 mg/litre. With S9 mix, there was a strong DNA-damaging effect, but, without S9 mix, a reverse effect was observed (Matsui et al., 1989).

8.6.1.5 Chromosomal effects

Rat liver (RL_1) cells were exposed to culture medium containing *cis*-1,3-dichloropropene (99.9%) in DMSO, at concentrations of 2.5, 5.0, or 10 µg/ml. No indication was found that the compound induced chromosome damage in the liver cells (Meyer, 1980).

The clastogenic potential of *trans*-1,3-dichloropropene (95.4% *trans*-isomer and 0.3% *cis*-isomer) was assessed from assays designed to monitor chromosome damage in CHO cells. Cultures were grown in incubated medium containing the test compound, for either 3 h in the presence of S9-mix (concentration 0, 0.5, 2.5 or 5.0 µg/ml) or 24 h in the absence of S9 mix (concentration 0, 3, 15 or 30 µg/ml). Methyl methane sulfonate and cyclophosphamide were used as positive controls. Metaphase cells were used for the analysis of chromosome aberrations after 8, 12, and 24 h, in the case of cultures with S9 mix, and, after 24 h, in the case of the cultures without S9 mix. At the 24-h sample time, it was concluded that *trans*-1,3-dichloropropene induced chromosome damage (gaps, breaks, and exchange figures) in the presence of S9 mix, but no effect was seen in its absence (Brooks & Wiggins, 1989b).

Loveday et al. (1989) tested 1,3-dichloropropene (97.1%) for its ability to induce chromosomal aberrations in cultured CHO cells. In the first study, without S9, 49.1 µg/ml produced a strong positive response, i.e., 16% of cells with aberrations (large number of gaps). No metaphase cells were seen at the 98.0 µg/ml dose level. In a repeat study, these results could not be confirmed with 50, 75, and 100 µg/ml. All 3 doses produced 50% decreases in cell confluency. When the compound was tested with S9 mix, no chromosomal aberrations were found at 50 µg/ml, the highest dose at which metaphase cells could be found.

Brooks & Wiggins (1991) assessed the mutagenic activity of cis-1,3-dichloropropene (94.5-97.5% cis-isomer, 1.5% trans-isomer, 0.25% 1,2-dichloropropane), in Chinese hamster ovary cells. The cultures were grown in medium containing the test substance for either 3 h in the presence of S9 mix or 24 h in the absence of S9 mix. Metaphase cells were prepared for analysis for chromosome aberrations, 24 h following initiation of exposure with, and without, S9 mix. From the data obtained at the 24-h sample time, it was concluded that cis-1,3-dichloropropene at 1, 5, or 10 µg/ml induced chromosome damage (gaps, breaks, and exchange figures) in the presence of S9 mix. No increase in metaphase chromosome damage was found with doses of up to 10 µg/ml in the absence of S9 mix.

Loveday et al. (1989) tested 1,3-dichloropropene (97.1%) for its ability to induce Sister Chromatid Exchanges (SCEs), in cultured Chinese hamster ovary cells. The test was carried out with, and without, rat liver S9 fraction. DMSO was used as the solvent. 1,3-Dichloropropene induced SCEs without S9 at a dose level of 29.9 µg/ml. A positive response was also found with S9.

Von der Hude et al. (1987) used the Sister Chromatid Exchange (SCE) test *in vitro* in Chinese hamster V79 cells without S9 mix, to evaluate the effect of 1,3-dichloropropene (80%). The concentrations tested were 0 (DMSO), and 0.1 up to 0.8 mmol/litre. The 0.8 mmol/litre dose was toxic to the cells. A dose-related increase in the number of SCEs was found. Negative results were obtained with S9, at dose levels of 0.1-3.3 mmol/litre.

8.6.2 In vivo *studies*

Telone II (49.5% cis- and 42.6% trans-1,3-dichloropropene) was evaluated in a mouse bone marrow micronucleus test to detect chromosomal aberrations and spindle malfunction. The substance (dissolved in corn oil) was administered to CD-1 (ICR) BR mice by single oral gavage at dose levels of 0 (corn oil), 38, 115, or 380 mg/kg body weight. Groups of animals were sacrificed at intervals of 24 and 48 h. A positive control group received cyclophosphamide at a dose of 120 mg/kg. There were no significant increases in the frequencies of micronucleated polychromatic erythrocytes in the Telone II groups compared with the controls. Positive results were obtained with the positive control group. Telone II was considered negative in the mouse bone marrow micronucleus test (Gollapudi et al., 1985).

Valencia et al. (1985) tested 1,3-dichloropropene (95.5%) for mutagenicity in *Drosophila melanogaster*. The compound was tested for the induction of sex-linked recessive lethals (SLRLs) by feeding the substance in a 5% aqueous sucrose solution. The dose level fed was 0 or 5750 mg/litre. The mortality rate was 33% and sterility 10%. 1,3-Dichloropropene induced an increased number of SLRLs, but no reciprocal translocations were induced.

The results of both dominant lethal and host-mediated assays carried out with "MIX D/D" were negative (see "Mixtures of dichloropropenes and dichloropropane", section 8.6.2).

8.6.3 Appraisal

1,3-Dichloropropene (*cis*- and *trans*-isomer) showed mutagenic activity in *Salmonella typhimurium*, especially in strains TA100 and TA1535 with, and without, metabolic activation. There is a difference in mutagenic potential between the *cis*- and *trans*-isomers in TA100 with, and without, activation. The *cis*-isomer induces a greater number of revertants than the *trans*-isomer.

1,3-Dichloropropene does not possess a genotoxic potential in a variety of non-bacterial studies. Gene mutation has not been detected in *in vitro* assays using the eukaryotic cell lines of either V79 or CHO (HGRPT locus) (Meyer, 1980; Mendrala, 1986). Chromosomal damage has not been observed *in vitro* with rat liver cell cultures or in an *in vivo* mouse micronucleus study using single oral doses of up to 380 mg/kg (Gollapudi et al., 1985). Interaction with DNA was not observed, even at cytotoxic doses, in an *in vitro* rat liver unscheduled DNA synthesis study (Mendrala, 1985). However, Schiffmann et al. (1983) found liver unscheduled DNA synthesis in Hela S3 cells.

8.7 Carcinogenicity

8.7.1 Oral

8.7.1.1 Mouse

A carcinogenicity study was carried out on groups of 50 male and 50 female (4-6 weeks old) $B_6C_3F_1$ mice at dose levels of 0, 50, or 100 mg (stabilized technical grade 1,3-dichloropropene)/kg body weight, administered in corn oil (5 ml/kg body weight), by gavage, 3 times per week for 104 weeks.

The technical product contained 41.6% *cis*- and 45.9% *trans*-isomer of 1,3-dichloropropene, 2.5% 1,2-dichloropropane, 1.5% trichloropropene isomer, nine other impurities, (7.5%) and epichlorohydrin 1% (as stabilizer). The initial mean body weights of the treated mice were lower (6-22%) than those of the controls. These differences were caused by failure to fully randomize the distribution of the animals. No clinical signs were observed. However, the survival of vehicle control male mice was significantly lower than that in either dose group. Thirty-nine control male mice died with myocarditis, 25, between weeks 48 and 51. A slight increase in mortality was found in the female mice at a dose level of 100 mg/kg body weight.

The reduced survival of the control male mice did not allow for an adequate evaluation of carcinogenicity in males in this study. But, in both sexes, there was evidence for a 1,3-dichloropropene-related increase in transitional cell carcinomas of the urinary bladder (without the presence of calculi), liver tumours, squamous cell papillomas and/or carcinomas of the forestomach, and of alveolar/bronchiolar adenomas and carcinomas of the lung, at 50 or 100 mg/kg body weight. In the female mice, an increase in basal cell or epithelial cell hyperplasia in the forestomach was also found (Table 14). It was stated that the presence of 1% epichlorohydrin, a direct acting mutagen and carcinogen (especially for the forestomach), may have influenced the development of forestomach lesions (Haseman et al., 1984; NTP, 1985; Yang, 1986; Yang et al., 1986).

8.7.1.2 Rat

A long-term carcinogenicity study was carried out on groups of 52 F344/N rats of each sex (aged 6 weeks), at dose levels of 0, 25, or 50 mg stabilized technical grade 1,3-dichloropropene/kg body weight, administered in corn oil (5 ml/kg body weight), by gavage, 3 times per week for 104 weeks.

The technical product contained 41.6% *cis*- and 45.9% *trans*-isomer of 1,3-dichloropropene, 2.5% 1,2-dichloropropane, 1.5% trichloropropene isomer, 9 other impurities, (7.5%) and epichlorohydrin 1% (as stabilizer). Additional groups of 25 rats of each sex were assigned to each dose group. At 9, 16, 21, 24, and 27 months of dosing, 5 rats/sex per group were killed and organs and tissues studied microscopically. Haematological and clinical-chemical studies were carried out on groups of 20 rats of each sex, 11-13 times in the first 70 weeks of the study. The mean body

Table 14. Occurrence of microscopic lesions in mice in a 2-year gavage study of 1,3-dichloropropene[a]

Lesions	Vehicle control		50 mg/kg body weight		100 mg/kg body weight	
	male	female	male	female	male	female
Urinary bladder						
Epithelial hyperplasia	[b]	2/50 (4%)	9/50 (18%)	15/50 (30%)	18/50 (36%)	19/48 (40%)
Transitional cell carcinoma	[b]	0/50 (0%)	0/50 (0%)	8/50 (16%)	2/50 (4%)	21/48 (44%)
Lung						
Alveolar/bronchiolar adenoma or carcinoma	1/50[c]	2/50 (4%)	13/50 (26%)	4/50 (8%)	12/50 (24%)	8/50 (16%)[*]
Forestomach						
Epithelial hyperplasia	[b]	1/50 (2%)	0/50 (0%)	1/50 (2%)	4/50 (8%)	21/50 (42%)[*]
Squamous cell papilloma or carcinoma	[b]	0/50 (0%)	2/50 (4%)	1/50 (2%)	3/50 (6%)[d]	4/50 (8%)[*]
Liver						
Hepatocellular adenoma or carcinoma	5/50[b]	1/50 (2%)	7/50 (14%)	8/50 (16%)[*]	13/50 (26%)	3/50 (6%)
Kidneys						
Hydronephrosis	[b]	0/50 (0%)	0/50 (0%)	2/50 (4%)	0/50 (0%)	14/50 (28%)

[a] From: NTP (1985).
[b] Too many animals died during the study, but no epithelial hyperplasia or neoplasia were observed in these animals.
[c] As [b] but, a lung adenoma was found in one animal.
[d] Only squamous cell papilloma.
[*] $P = \leq 0.05$.

weight of high-dose male rats was about 5% lower than those of the control and low-dose rats. No differences in body weight were observed in female animals. Mortality was comparable with the controls. The primary organs affected were the forestomach and liver. The incidences of non-neoplastic and neoplastic lesions are summarized in Table 15.

Under the conditions of the study, 1,3-dichloropropene induced an increased incidence of squamous cell papillomas and carcinomas of the forestomach. In addition, a dose-related trend was observed in the incidence of neoplastic nodules in the livers of male rats. It was stated that the presence of 1% epichlorohydrin, a direct acting mutagen and carcinogen (especially for the forestomach), may have influenced the development of forestomach lesions (Haseman et al., 1984; NTP, 1985; Yang, 1986; Yang et al., 1986).

In the ancillary study, dose-related lesions were observed in the forestomach and liver. The development of the forestomach basal-cell hyperplasia and squamous-cell papilloma followed a time-dependent trend in high-dose males and females. Basal-cell hyperplasia was seen 9-16 months after dosing started. The neoplasms of the forestomach and liver were not seen until 24 months after dosing began.

8.7.2 Inhalation

8.7.2.1 Mouse

Groups of 50 male and 50 female $B_6C_3F_1$ mice (6-7 weeks of age) were exposed to 1,3-dichloropropene for 6 h/day, 5 days per week for up to 24 months. In addition, 2 ancillary groups, each with 10 animals/sex per exposure level, were exposed to 1,3-dichloropropene for 6 or 12 months. The mice were exposed to 1,3-dichloropropane vapour at 0, 22.7, 90.8, or 272 mg/m^3. The composition of the technical-grade 1,3-dichloropropene was 1,3-dichloropropene 92.1% (*cis*-49.5% and *trans* 42.6%); 1,2-dichloropropane 0.7%; and 5.2% mixtures of hexanes and hexadienes. Epoxidized soybean oil (approximately 2%) was added as stabilizing agent. Besides body weights, clinical-chemical parameters in the blood and urine and haematological parameters were determined for all animals terminated at 6 and 12 months and for 20 animals/sex per group at 24 months. At 6, 12, and 24 months, animals were sacrificed and the weight of 5 organs determined; a large number of organs and tissues were examined histopathologically.

Table 15. Occurrence of microscopic lesions in rats in a 2-year gavage study of 1,3-dichloropropene[a]

Lesions	Vehicle control		50 mg/kg body weight		100 mg/kg body weight	
	male	female	male	female	male	female
Forestomach						
Epithelial hyperplasia	2/52 (4%)	1/52 (2%)	5/52 (10%)	0/52 (0%)	13/52 (25%)[c]	16/52 (31%)[c]
Squamous cell papilloma or carcinoma	1/52 (2%)	0/52 (0%)	1/52 (2%)	2/52 (4%)[b]	13/52 (25%)[c]	3/52 (6%)[b]
Liver						
Neoplastic nodule or carcinoma	1/52 (2%)	6/52 (12%)	6/52 (12%)[c]	6/52 (12%)[c]	7/52 (13%)[c]	10/52 (19%)

[a] From: NTP (1985).
[b] Only squamous cell papilloma.
[c] $P = \leq 0.05$

No significant differences in survival rates were observed between the groups. The body weights of male mice exposed to 272 mg 1,3-dichloropropene/m^3 were statistically significantly depressed in comparison with the controls. Examination of haematological and clinical-chemical parameters and urinalysis did not indicate any toxicity resulting from exposure to 1,3-dichloropropene for 6, 12, or 24 months.

The mean relative liver weight of male animals exposed to 272 mg/m^3 showed a statistically significant decrease. Gross patho-logical examination of mice revealed morphological alterations involving the urinary bladder and lung, which were attributed to exposure to 1,3-dichloropropene. The bladder mucosal surface in females exposed to 272 mg/m^3 for 12 months and 90.8 and 272 mg/m^3 for 24 months had a roughened appearance. In addition, a statistically significantly increased number of the females exposed to 90.8 and 272 mg/m^3 showed inflammation and epithelial hyperplasia of the bladder mucosa, after 24 months. An increased number of male animals exposed to 272 mg/m^3 also showed inflammation.

Female mice exposed to 90.8 or 272 mg/m^3 and males exposed to 272 mg/m^3 showed hypertrophy and hyperplasia of the nasal epithelium and degeneration of the olfactory epithelium. Additional microscopic changes, considered exposure-related, were hyperplasia and hyperkeratosis in the forestomach of 8/50 male mice following 24 months exposure to 272 mg/m^3. A statistically significant increase in the incidence of a benign tumour, bronchio-alveolar adenoma, was observed in male mice exposed to 272 mg 1,3-dichloropropene vapour/m^3 for 24 months [22/50 (44%) vs 9/50 (18%) in controls]. No statistically significant increase in tumour incidence was found in the groups exposed to 1,3-dichloropropene at 22.7 and 90.8 mg/m^3 (Table 16). The incidence of lung tumours in the males exposed to 272 mg/m^3 was somewhat higher (7-32%) than the range of historical control values for this type of tumour in male $B_6C_3F_1$ mice in 7 previous, long-term studies. The NOAEL in this study on mice for hypertrophy/hyperplasia of the nasal epithelium was 22.7 mg/m^3 (Yano et al., 1985; Stott et al., 1987; Lomax et al., 1989).

8.7.2.2 Rat

Groups of 50 male and 50 female Fischer 344 rats (7-9 weeks of age) were exposed to 1,3-dichloropropene for 6 h/day, 5 days/week for up to 24 months. In addition, 2 ancillary groups,

Table 16. Incidence of various types of lesions observed in a mouse inhalation study with 1,3-dichloropropene[a]

	Males (mg/m^3)				Females (mg/m^3)			
	0	22.7	90.8	272	0	22.7	90.8	272
Urinary bladder								
Hyperplasia mucosa (simple or nodular)	4/48 (9%)	7/48 (15%)	11/48 (23%)	37/47 (79%)[b]	1/47 (2%)	4/46 (9%)	21/48 (44%)[b]	44/45 (98%)[b]
Lungs								
Bronchio-alveolar adenoma	9/50 (18%)	6/50 (12%)	13/50 (26%)	22/50 (44%)[b]	4/50 (8%)	3/50 (6%)	5/50 (6%)	3/50 (6%)
Nasal tissues								
Degeneration of olfactory epithelium	1/50 (2%)	0/50	1/50 (2%)	48/50 (96%)[b]	0/50	0/50	1/50 (2%)	45/50 (90%)[b]
Hyperplasia and hypertrophy of respiratory epithelium	5/50 (10%)	1/50 (2%)	4/50 (8%)	48/50 (96%)[b]	4/50 (8%)	4/50 (8%)	28/50 (56%)[b]	49/50 (98%)[b]
Stomach								
Squamous papilloma	0/50 (0%)	3/50 (6%)	2/50 (4%)	0/50 (0%)	3/50 (6%)	2/50 (4%)	0/50 (0%)	3/50 (6%)

[a] From: Lomax et al. (1989).
[b] Statistical difference from control mean identified by using Yate's χ^2 pairwise test, $\alpha = 0.05$.

each comprising 10 animals/sex per exposure level, were exposed to 1,3-dichloropropene for 6 or 12 months. The animals were exposed to 0, 22.7, 90.8, or 272 mg/m^3. The chemical composition of the test material was 92.1% 1,3-dichloropropene (*cis*-49.5% and *trans*-42.6%), 0.7% 1,2-dichloropropane, and mixtures of hexanes and hexadiens. Epoxidized soybean oil (approximately 2%) was present as stabilizer. Besides body weights of the animals, clinical-chemical parameters in the blood and urine and haematological parameters were determined for all animals terminated at 6 and 12 months and for 20 animals/sex from each exposure group at 24 months.

At 6, 12, or 24 months, animals were sacrificed and the weight of 5 organs determined; a large number of organs and tissues were examined histopathologically. No significant influence on survival was observed. Mean body weights of both male and female rats exposed to 272 mg/m^3 were statistically significantly decreased compared with mean control values. Examination of haematological and clinical-chemical parameters, urinalysis, and organ weights did not indicate any toxicity resulting from exposure to 1,3-dichloropropene for 6, 12, or 24 months.

Gross pathological examination did not indicate any exposure-related effects after 6, 12, or 24 months. Exposure-related histological effects occurred in nasal tissues of rats exposed to 272 mg/m^3 for 24 months (Table 17), but not for 6 or 12 months. The microscopic changes were located in the olfactory mucosa, which covers the upper portions of the nasal cavity, nasal septum, and turbinates. The changes were characterized by unilateral or bilateral decreased thickness of olfactory epithelium and fibrosis of the submucosal tissues underlying eroded olfactory epithelium. At the lower dose levels, females did not show histopathological changes in the nasal tissue, while one male exposed to 22.7 mg/m^3 and one exposed to 90.8 mg/m^3 showed decreased thickness of the olfactory epithelium. No effects were seen in the controls. No statistically significant increase in tumour incidence was found in exposed rats compared with controls (Lomax et al., 1987, 1989).

8.7.3 Appraisal

Exposure to 1,3-dichloropropene, through inhalation, for up to 24 months did not have any demonstrable effects on survival or spontaneous tumour development in male and female Fischer 344 rats. In mice, an increased incidence of bronchio-alveolar adenomas was found in the lungs of male mice, exposed to

Table 17. Microscopic changes in the nasal tissues of rats exposed to Telone II at 272 mg/m³[a]

Microscopic change	Vehicle control (male and female)	Overall incidence	
		Male	Female
Decreased thickness of olfactory epithelium	0/100	20/50[b] (40%)	15/50[b] (31%)
Erosion of olfactory epithelium	0/100	15/50[b] (30%)	6/50 (12%)
Submucosal fibrosis	0/100	6/50[b] (12%)	2/50 (4%)

[a] From: Lomax et al. (1989).
[b] Statistical difference identified from control mean of Yate's χ^2 pairwise test, $\alpha = 0.05$.

272 mg/m³, but not at the lower dose level (90.8 mg/m³). The oral gavage study with 1,3-dichloropropene demonstrated an increased incidence of forestomach neoplasms in rats of both sexes at dose levels of 50 mg/kg body weight, administered 3 times/week for 24 months. Male rats treated with 25 or 50 mg/kg also had an increased incidence of neoplastic nodules in the liver.

In both the oral gavage and inhalation mouse bioassays with 1,3-dichloropropene, a tumorigenic response was noted in tissues with which 1,3-dichloropropene had direct contact, i.e., the stomach and the lung. However, in the gavage study, tumours were also induced at sites distant from that at the primary "portal-of-entry" (lung and urinary bladder). This was not the case in the inhalation study, despite the fact that the dose of 1,3-dichloropropene received on a mg/kg body weight per day basis by mice exposed for 5 days/week through inhalation was approximately 2-3 times higher than the dose levels administered orally 3 times/week in the NTP (1985). The degeneration and subsequent hyperplasia of nasal and forestomach epithelium occurred only at concentrations that are known to deplete glutathione levels in these tissues. Tumorigenic effects occur at doses higher than those causing glutathione depletion and tissue damage.

The same mouse strain and similar test materials relative to 1,3-dichloropropene were used in both bioassays, but there was a difference in the stabilizing agents in the test materials. The 1,3-dichloropropene used in the NTP study was stabilized with 1% epichlorohydrin, a carcinogen. It has been suggested that epichlorohydrin may have played a role in the tumorigenic response obtained in the gavage study because of the bolus nature of its administration. However, it is not known whether the increased incidence of tumours in the urinary bladder, lungs, forestomach, and liver in the mouse gavage study are attributable to the treatment with 1,3-dichloropropene or the effect of epichlorohydrin, since carcinogenicity studies of epichlorohydrin in mice have not been performed yet. In the inhalation study carried out by Lomax et al. (1989), the 1,3-dichloropropene was stabilized with the relatively nontoxic epoxidized soybean oil. The role of the stabilizing additive epichlorohydrin in generating the different tumours seen in the oral gavage studies on 1,3-dichloropropene is still uncertain. This question has to be further investigated before a more definite conclusion about the carcinogenic potential of 1,3-dichloropropene can be drawn.

8.7.4 Dermal and subcutaneous (mouse)

Groups of 30 female Ha:ICR Swiss strain mice (6-8 weeks old) were treated with 0.2 ml acetone containing 41 or 122 mg purified *cis*-1,3 dichloropropene, applied to shaven skin 3 times weekly, for approximately 18 months. Control mice received acetone. In the group treated with 41 mg, no papillomas were found, but at the 122 mg dose, 3 animals showed papillomas, and 2, carcinomas. No tumours were found at distant sites. *Cis*-1,3-dichloropropene, applied once on the skin at a dose of 122 mg/mouse, was followed after 14 days by the application of 5 μg phorbol myristate acetate in 0.2 ml acetone, 3 times weekly until the end of the study. No skin tumour-initiating activity was observed (van Duuren et al., 1979).

A group of 30 female Ha:ICR Swiss mice were given weekly subcutaneous injections in the left flank of 0.05 ml trioctanoin containing 3 mg purified *cis*-1,3-dichloropropene per injection. The study lasted 538 days. Control animals received only the vehicle. Six out of 30 mice showed local fibrosarcomas, whereas vehicle control animals did not. A positive control of 0.3 mg beta-propiolactone produced local sarcomas in 24 out of 30 mice during a 378-day period (van Duuren et al., 1979).

The relevance of the subcutaneous route for the assessment of carcinogenic properties remains questionable, especially when injections of an irritant material are made. It is probable that the persistent and physical properties rather than the chemical characteristics of *cis*-1,3-dichloropropene are responsible for production of local sarcomas.

8.8 Factors modifying toxicity, toxicity of metabolites, mode of action

8.8.1 Toxicity of the metabolites, cis- and trans-1,3-dichloropropene oxide

There is some evidence that a small proportion of *cis*-1,3-dichloropropene is metabolized to *cis*-1,3-dichloropropene oxide (Fig. 5; Hutson, 1984).

8.8.1.1 Mutagenicity

Cis- and *trans*-1,3-dichloropropene oxide were tested for mutagenicity, in the absence of metabolic activation, in *Salmonella typhimurium* TA1535 and *Escherichia coli* WP2 *uvr A*, and for preferential inhibition of growth of DNA-repair-polymerase-deficient *E. coli*. Both oxides were potent mutagens and DNA modifiers. In *Salmonella typhimurium* TA1535, treated with 0.025 μmol/ml and in *E. coli* WP2 *uvr A* treated with 0.05 μmol/ml of bacterial suspension, a significant increase in revertant colonies was found. A gene mutation test with *E. coli* (pol A_1^-/pol A_1^+) in the absence of metabolic activation, already showed an effect with 0.0005 μmol/ml (Kline et al., 1982).

In the absence of an S9-fraction, *cis*-dichloropropene oxide was strongly mutagenic towards *S. typhimurium* TA100. The mutagenicity reached a maximum at 25 μg/plate. Above 300 μg/plate, marked cytotoxicity was observed. Glutathione (5 mmol/litre) caused a significant inhibitory effect on the mutagenicity and cytotoxicity of this epoxide, but did not offer complete protection. Inclusion of glutathione (5 mmol/litre) together with S9-fraction afforded complete protection over the range of concentrations of *cis*-dichloropropene oxide up to 100 μg/plate (Hutson 1984; Watson et al., 1986a).

Cis- and *trans*-1,3-dichloropropene oxide were tested in a quantitative Syrian hamster embryo cell model. Both compounds at dose levels of 0.005, 0.01, or 0.02 mmol/litre (*cis*-isomer) and 0.01, 0.025, or 0.05 mmol/litre (*trans*-isomer) induced morphological transformation of the Syrian hamster embryo cells (DiPaolo & Doniger, 1982).

8.8.1.2 Carcinogenicity

Female ICR/Ha Swiss mice (30 per group) were treated 3 times weekly, with cis-1,3-dichloropropene oxide or trans-1,3-dichloropropene oxide (containing 10-15% of m-dichlorobenzene) on the skin. The dose level was 10 mg in 0.1 ml of acetone. The controls received only acetone. The median survival time was comparable with that of the controls (over 500 days). With cis-dichloropropene oxide, 16/30 mice had local papillomas and 10/30 squamous cell carcinomas of the skin; with trans-dichloropropene oxide, this was 20/30 and 17/30, respectively. No tumours were found in the control animals (van Duuren et al., 1983).

A study was also carried out on the same strain of mice using subcutaneous injections. Thirty female mice received 500 µg cis-dichloropropene oxide or trans-dichloropropene oxide in 0.05 ml tricaprylin once weekly. The median survival time was comparable to that of controls. With cis-dichloropropene oxide, 4 animals had a local (fibro)sarcoma and one carcinoma, and, with trans-dichloropropene oxide, 5 animals had fibrosarcomas. No tumours were found in the vehicle controls (van Duuren et al., 1983).

8.8.2 Role of oxidation

When purified cis-1,3-dichloropropene was heated for a few hours in an oxygen atmosphere, in either the light or dark, the non-mutagenic cis-1,3-dichloropropene became strongly mutagenic. Heating under nitrogen was negative. Storage of cis-1,3-dichloropropene at room temperature, in the presence of oxygen, for two months, made it mutagenic (Watson et al., 1987). Talcott & King (1984) demonstrated that purified samples of 1,3-dichloropropene were not mutagenic to *Salmonella typhimurium* TA100. Four preparations of 1,3-dichloropropene were separated into different fractions and analysed for mutagenic activity. The fraction containing polar metabolites was found to be mutagenic. Its composition was too complex to characterize completely, but 2 mutagens, epichlorohydrin and 1,3-dichloro-2-propanol, were identified.

Watson et al. (1986 a,b; 1987) confirmed that the direct mutagenicity, inducing base-pair mutations, previously observed in *Salmonella typhimurium* TA100 treated with cis-1,3-dichloropropene, was caused by trace impurities. These impurities resulted from the autooxidation of cis- and trans-1,3-dichloropropene and were identified as cis- and trans-dichloropropene oxides. The dichloropropene oxides made a significant contribution towards the intrinsic mutagenicity, when tested in *S. typhimurium* TA100 (see section 8.8.1.1).

The proposed formation of *cis*- and *trans*-dichloropropene oxides is shown in Fig. 6.

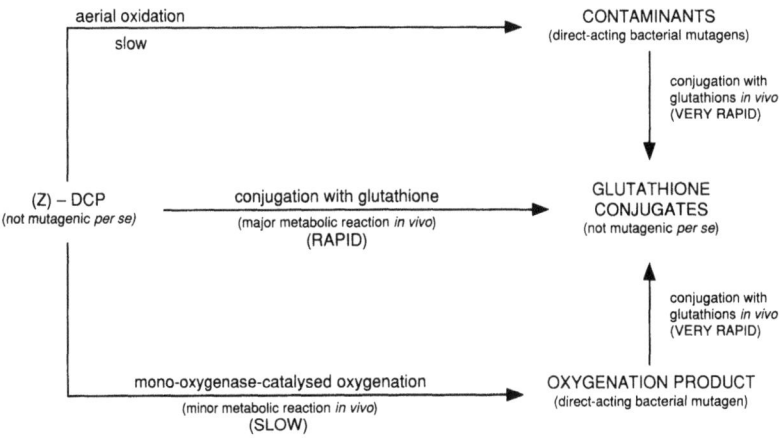

Fig. 6. Proposed mechanism of autooxidation of cis-1,3-dichloropropene. From: Watson et al. (1987).

Autooxidation of *cis*-1,3-dichloropropene occurs after radical initiation (5) to give the alkyl peroxy radical (6), which reacts with a second molecule of *cis*-1,3-dichloropropene to give the free radical intermediate (7). Free rotation can occur in this molecule, prior to expulsion of the alkoxy radical (8), with concomitant formation of both *cis*- and *trans*-dichloropropene oxides (3) and (4). The alkoxy radical (8) may further abstract a proton or chlorine from *cis*-1,3-dichloropropene, thus, continuing the chain reaction. Autooxidation reactions often proceed via several pathways and in the case of *cis*-dichloropropene there are minor products, such as a 2-hydroxyperoxy intermediate, and unstable 1,2-dioxetanes leading to 1,3-dichloro-2-propanol and aldehydes, respectively. *Trans*-dichloropropene was considerably more resistant to autooxidations than *cis*-dichloropropene (Watson et al., 1987).

8.8.3 Role of glutathione

Glutathione (GSH) at physiological concentrations in *in vitro* bacterial test systems of *Salmonella typhimurium* TA100 has been shown to have a protective effect, i.e., a virtual elimination of the mutagenic response to 1,3-dichloropropene (Hutson & Stoydin, 1977; DeLorenzo et al., 1977; Brooks et al., 1978; Climie et al., 1979; Wright & Creedy, 1982; Creedy & Hutson, 1982).

This protective effect occurs in either the absence or the presence of S9 for both the *cis*- and *trans*-isomer. In the absence of a rat liver fraction, the chemical reaction of *cis*-1,3-dichloropropene with glutathione is slow, and, in the presence of the rat liver fraction, the reaction is rapid due to enzyme catalysis. The *trans*-isomer (in the presence of the *cis* compound) was degraded 4-5 times more slowly than the *cis*-isomer (Hutson & Stoydin, 1977; Climie et al., 1979).

This protective effect in the presence of S9 is consistent with the operation of a glutathione transferase enzyme occurring in the added S9 fraction. This enzyme, which conjugates *cis*-1,3-dichloropropene with glutathione, is also present in mammalian cells and the metabolic studies have shown that it plays a key role in the rapid detoxification of *cis*-1,3-dichloropropene in mammalian tissue (Climie et al., 1979; Brooks & Wiggins, 1991).

There is some evidence that the mutagenicity of these preparations is due to contaminants and that the protective action of glutathione is due to spontaneous conjugation reactions between these contaminants and glutathione. Pure *cis*-dichloropropene did undergo metabolic activation catalysed by microsomal monooxygenase system from the rat liver. Thus, a small, but significant, dose-dependent increase in mutation was observed when *cis*-dichloropropene was tested in *S. typhimurium* TA100, in the presence of S9-liver fraction. When this S9 fraction was replaced by washed microsomes, which remove the glutathione activity, the mutagenic effect of *cis*-1,3-dichloropropene was increased. Replacement of the glutathione *S*-alkyl transferase(s) in the microsomal fraction from an S100 fraction, restored the glutathione-conjugating activity and afforded complete protection against *cis*-1,3-dichloropropene. *Cis*-dichloropropene undergoes rapid conjugation with glutathione in the presence of the mentioned transferase(s), which limits the availability of *cis*-dichloropropene to undergo mono-oxygenase-catalysed bioactivation. These results also provide some evidence that these glutathione-linked conjugation systems also afford efficient protection against the mutagenic hazard posed by the bioactivation products of *cis*-dichloropropene. Thus, the microbial mutagenicity of *cis*-dichloropropene oxide was significantly reduced by glutathione (5 mmol/litre) and this protective action was strongly enhanced in the presence of glutathione *S*-alkyl transferases from the S100 (Fig. 7).

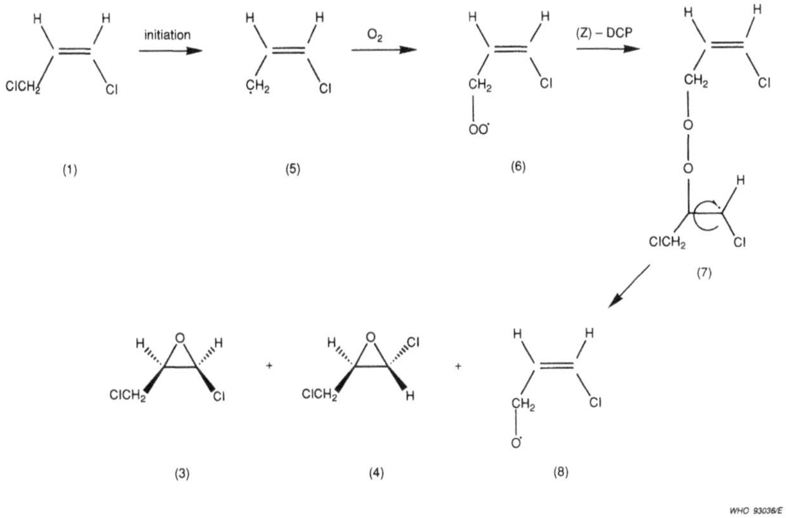

Fig. 7. Relationship of oxidation, bioactivation, and conjunction pathways of *cis*-dichloropropene. From: Watson et al. (1986b, 1987).

It was concluded that the degree to which the genotoxic potential of *cis*-dichloropropene or its autooxidation products is expressed *in vivo* is likely to be lower than that found by microbial mutation assays. *Cis*-dichloropropene is efficiently detoxified in mammals by the operation of a glutathione-dependent *S*-alkyl transferase (Watson et al., 1987).

8.8.4 Effect on liver enzyme activity

Miyaoka et al. (1990) studied the mechanism of 1,3-dichloropropene-induced hepatotoxicity in male mice of the ICR strain (6 weeks old). 1,3-Dichloropropene (300 mg/kg body weight), administered by gavage in corn oil, increased plasma GOT and GPT activities significantly, and centrilobular swelling occurred in the liver, 15 h after treatment. No such effect was found with 100 mg/kg body weight. Pretreatment of piperonylbutoxide (PIB, a cytochrome P450 inhibitor), at 200 mg/kg body weight i.p., significantly suppressed the elevation of plasma GOT and GPT activities caused by 300 mg 1,3-dichloropropene/kg body weight, but increased the 1,3-dichloropropene concentration in the liver. The PIB pretreatment decreased the cytochrome P450 contents in liver microsomes, but prevented further reduction of cytochrome P450 after 1,3-dichloropropene treatment.

With pretreatment with L-buthionine-S,R sulfoximine (a GSH depleting agent) at 1600 mg/kg body weight, plasma GOT activities increased significantly in animals receiving 100 mg 1,3-dichloropropene, whereas liver GSH contents and GST activity decreased. Cysteine administration, 2 h after 1,3-dichloropropene treatment, did not decrease the cytochrome P450 content, though it prevented the elevation of GOT and GPT activities and increased hepatic GSH concentration. The results suggest that 1,3-dichloropropene is biotransformed via cytochrome P450, and that the metabolites induce liver damage. GSH plays an important role in the detoxification of 1,3-dichloropropene (Miyaoka et al., 1990).

9. EFFECTS ON HUMANS

9.1 General population

9.1.1 Acute toxicity - poisoning incidents

In a truck accident in California in 1975, about 4500 litres of 1,3-dichloropropene (92%) was slowly spilled on to the highway. An estimated 80 persons were exposed to the vapour. Forty-six persons were examined at hospitals. The following symptoms were found in a small number of persons (4-6), headache, vomiting and nausea, dizziness, irritation of mucous membranes, and chest discomfort. Three persons lost consciousness at the scene of the accident. In 11 out of 41 persons, slightly elevated SGOT and/or SGPT values were found. Twenty-eight patients were interviewed 1 or 2 weeks later. The most common symptoms were: headache (12), abdominal discomfort (6), chest discomfort (5), and malaise (5). Twenty-one patients were interviewed after 2 years; 10 patients complained of severe or unusual headache, 10 of chest pain or discomfort, and 13 of "personality changes" (fatigue, irritability, difficulty in concentrating, or decreased libido). The frequency of these long-persisting symptoms was not associated with the intensity of the exposure (Flessel et al., 1978).

Markovitz & Crosby (1984) reported 9 cases of acute poisoning following accidental over-exposure to 1,3-dichloropropene. The chemical spilled as the driver jack-knifed the container. Two of these cases died 6 years later, due to diffuse histocytic lymphoma. Authors have reported another case of myelo-monocytic leukaemia where the patient had been accidentally over-exposed to 1,3-dichloropropene (see section 9.2.2).

9.1.2 Controlled human studies

A smell detection test with 10 human volunteers was carried out. A level of 13.6 mg 1,3-dichloropropene/m^3 air was detected by 7 out of 10 volunteers. Some reported that the sense of smell diminished after a few minutes. Even a level of 4.54 mg/m^3 was detected by these 7 persons, but it was noticeably fainter than 13.6 mg/m^3 (Torkelson & Oyen, 1977).

In a study designed to determine the odour threshold of Telone II among 22 individuals, the lowest concentration at which odour was detected was 20 ± 14 mg/m^3. This level is slightly above the

US threshold limit value time-weighted average of 4.54 mg/m^3, but below the short-term exposure limit of 45.4 mg/m^3 (Rick & McCarty, 1988).

9.2 Occupational exposure

9.2.1 General

The most likely routes of human exposure to 1,3-dichloropropene are through inhalation and the skin. Irritation of the eyes and upper respiratory mucosa, accompanied by lacrimation, appear promptly after exposure to vapours (Gosselin et al., 1976).

Inhalation by humans of air containing concentrations greater than 6810 mg/m^3 produces headaches, mucous membrane irritation, dizziness, nausea, vomiting, gasping, coughing, substernal pain, and respiratory distress (Gosselin et al., 1976; Flessel et al., 1978). Lower concentrations produce central nervous system depression and moderate irritation of the respiratory system.

A 44-year-old male process operator at a pesticide plant had acute bullous dermatitis on both feet in 1988. Approximately one year later, an identical dermatitis developed. In both periods, he contaminated his shoes with a 1,3-dichloropropene formulation (D-D-95). In a patch test with 1,3-dichloropropene, even a concentration of 0.005% produced a positive reaction. Twenty volunteers did not react in this patch test at a concentration of 0.05% (Bousema et al., 1991).

Maddy et al. (1990) summarized the pesticides that caused occupational illness/injury, reported by physicians in California during 1987. 1,3-Dichloropropene caused one case of systemic illness in that period. In the year 1986, 3 cases were mentioned, one with systemic effects, one with skin effects, and one with eye injury (Edmiston & Maddy, 1987).

Fifteen applicators of 1,3-dichloropropene were studied for personal air exposure, urinary excretion of the metabolite, and excretion of the renal tubular enzyme N-acetyl glucosaminidase (NAG). Each was studied for four, 6-8 h consecutive intervals following base-line determinations. The duration of exposure ranged from 120 to 697 min and the personal air concentrations ranged from 0.3 to 9.4 mg/m^3. The 24-h urinary excretion of the metabolite (average 2.6 mg, range: 0.5-9.2 mg) correlated well with the 1,3-dichloropropene air exposure product (minutes exposed × mg/m^3). The mean excretion of NAG for all intervals was 2.6 mU/mg of creatinine (range: 1.0-7.7 mU/mg of creatinine); in 24 h, the mean was 4940 mU with a range of 278-8956 mU. Four of the 15 workers had an NAG activity of > 4 mU/mg creatinine in any of their urine collected after the base line. Nine workers showed increases in NAG excretion of more than 25% compared with the base line. The authors concluded that the elevated excretion of NAG indicated a possible subclinical nephrotoxic effect in the workers, though no complaints or cases of renal injury were reported (Osterloh et al., 1989). Stott et al. (1990) commented that the slight increase in NAG in the urine might be a result of the stimulation of exocytosis or an increase (induction) in the NAG activity in the kidneys, rather than an indication of nephrotoxicity. Taken together with the known metabolism and toxicity of 1,3-dichloropropene in laboratory animals, the findings by Osterloh et al. (1989) do not suggest any untoward effects in workers exposed occupationally to low levels of 1,3-dichloropropene.

Fourteen workers applying 1,3-dichloropropene were monitored at the start of the season, in July, and at the end of the season, in October, for liver function. The following parameters were measured; alanine aminotransferase, aspartate aminotransferase, alkaline phosphatase, lactic dehydrogenase, gamma-glutamyltranspeptidase, and total bilirubin. Total bilirubin was significantly decreased at the end of the season. In combination with an increase in serum gamma-glutamyltranspeptidase activity this indicates moderate hepatic enzyme induction. The renal function was also studied by measuring creatinine and beta-2-microglobulin in serum and beta-2-microglobulin, albumin, alanine-aminopeptidase, beta-galactosidase, and retinol-binding protein in urine. The glomerular function parameters (increased albumin in urine and decreased creatinine in serum) changed significantly during the season. The tubular function (retinol-binding protein) also increased. On the basis of these data, a subclinical nephrotoxic effect cannot be excluded. Effects on the glutathione conjugation capacity were studied by measuring erythrocyte glutathione-S-transferase activity and blood glutathione concentration. Both parameters were significantly decreased (Brouwer et al., 1991b). The cause-effect relationship with 1,3-dichloropropene exposure has been questioned (Van Sittert et al., 1991).

9.2.2 Acute toxicity - poisoning incidents

A farmer in good health developed pain in the right ear, nasal mucosa, and pharynx after applying 1,3-dichloropropene to his fields from his tractor for 30 days. Hospital examination showed a red and painful external ear, hyperaemia, and superficial ulcerations of the nasal mucosa, and inflammation of the pharynx. The hose containing the 1,3-dichloropropene had a small leak, which had sprayed the chemical near the right side of his face. Over the following year, the man developed myelo-monocytic leukaemia. The man died of pneumonia 5 weeks after entering the hospital (Markovitz & Crosby, 1984; NTP, 1985; Yang, 1986). The Task Group considers that the cause-effect relationship in this case is doubtful.

9.2.3 Effects of short- and long-term exposure

The fertility status of 63 males employed in the production of chlorinated three-carbon compounds were investigated in comparison with 63 non-exposed persons (at least 5 years without exposure). Data from reproductive medical history, hormone determination, and semen analysis were used. There were no indications for an association between lowered fertility by the standard fertility parameters, and exposure to allyl chloride, epichlorohydrin, and 1,3-dichloropropene in the quantities occurring in the working environment. A possible source of bias in this study stems from the relatively low (64%) volunteer rate from the exposed group and the lack of an estimate of the individual variation (Venable et al., 1980).

10. PREVIOUS EVALUATIONS BY INTERNATIONAL BODIES

1,3-Dichloropropene (technical grade) was considered by working groups of the International Agency for Research on Cancer (IARC) in 1986 (IARC, 1986) and 1987 (IARC,1987). In the updating of 1987, it was evaluated as follows. "There is sufficient evidence for the carcinogenicity of 1,3-dichloropropene (technical-grade) in experimental animals. There is inadequate evidence for the carcinogenicity of 1,3-dichloropropene (technical-grade) in humans. The agent is possibly carcinogenic to humans (Group 2B)".

Based on the results from 2-year gavage studies on rats and mice, using the linearized multistage model, the drinking-water concentration for an excess life-time cancer risk of 10^4, 10^5, or 10^6 is estimated to be 20, 2.0, or 0.2 µg/litre, respectively (WHO/EURO, 1990).

PART B

ENVIRONMENTAL HEALTH CRITERIA

FOR

1,2-DICHLOROPROPANE

CONTENTS

ENVIRONMENTAL HEALTH CRITERIA FOR
1,2-DICHLOROPROPANE

1. SUMMARY AND EVALUATION, CONCLUSIONS AND
   RECOMMENDATIONS   123

   1.1 Summary and evaluation   123
       1.1.1 Use, environmental fate, and
             environmental levels   123
       1.1.2 Kinetics and metabolism   124
       1.1.3 Effects on organisms in the environment   124
       1.1.4 Effects on experimental animals and
             in vitro test systems   125
       1.1.5 Effects on human beings   126
   1.2 Conclusions   127
   1.3 Recommendations   127

2. IDENTITY, PHYSICAL AND CHEMICAL PROPERTIES,
   ANALYTICAL METHODS   128

   2.1 Identity   128
   2.2 Physical and chemical properties   128
   2.3 Conversion factors   128
   2.4 Analytical methods   129

3. SOURCES OF HUMAN AND ENVIRONMENTAL
   EXPOSURE   130

   3.1 Natural occurrence   130
   3.2 Man-made sources   130
   3.3 Uses   130

4. ENVIRONMENTAL TRANSPORT, DISTRIBUTION, AND
   TRANSFORMATION   131

   4.1 Transport and distribution between media   131
       4.1.1 Air   131
       4.1.2 Soil   131
             4.1.2.1 Volatilization   131
             4.1.2.2 Uptake in crops   131
             4.1.2.3 Movement in soil   132
   4.2 Biotransformation   132
   4.3 Bioconcentration   132

5.	ENVIRONMENTAL LEVELS AND HUMAN EXPOSURE		133
	5.1 Environmental levels		133
	5.1.1	Air	133
	5.1.2	Water and soil	133
	5.1.3	Crops	135
6.	KINETICS AND METABOLISM		136
	6.1 Absorption, distribution, and elimination		136
	6.1.1	Oral	136
	6.1.2	Inhalation	137
	6.1.3	Intraperitoneal	137
	6.2 Metabolic transformation		138
7.	EFFECTS ON ORGANISMS IN THE ENVIRONMENT		141
	7.1 Aquatic organisms		141
	7.1.1	Algae	141
	7.1.2	Invertebrates	141
	7.1.3	Fish	142
		7.1.3.1 Acute toxicity	142
		7.1.3.2 Short-term/long-term toxicity	142
	7.2 Terrestrial organisms		142
	7.2.1	Earthworms	142
	7.2.2	Plants	142
8.	EFFECTS ON EXPERIMENTAL ANIMALS AND *IN VITRO* TEST SYSTEMS		144
	8.1 Single exposures		144
	8.2 Short-term exposures		144
	8.2.1	Oral	144
		8.2.1.1 Mouse	144
		8.2.1.2 Rat	144
	8.2.2	Inhalation	146
		8.2.2.1 Mouse	146
		8.2.2.2 Rat	146
		8.2.2.3 Rabbit	147
	8.3 Reproduction, embryotoxicity, and teratogenicity		147
	8.3.1	Reproduction	147
	8.3.2	Teratogenicity	148
		8.3.2.1 Oral (rat)	148
		8.3.2.2 Oral (rabbit)	148
	8.4 Mutagenicity and related end-points		149

		8.4.1	*In vitro* studies	149
			8.4.1.1 Microorganisms	149
			8.4.1.2 Mammalian cells	149
		8.4.2	*In vivo* studies	152
			8.4.2.1 *Drosophila melanogaster*	152
			8.4.2.2 Dominant lethal test	152
			8.4.2.3 Miscellaneous	153
	8.5	Carcinogenicity		153
		8.5.1	Oral (mouse)	153
		8.5.2	Oral (rat)	154
	8.6	Factors modifying toxicity		155
	8.7	Special studies		156
		8.7.1	Liver	156
		8.7.2	Kidneys	157
		8.7.3	Central nervous system	158
9.	EFFECTS ON HUMANS			160
	9.1	General population exposure		160
		9.1.1	Acute toxicity - poisoning incidents	160
	9.2	Occupational exposure		160
10.	PREVIOUS EVALUATIONS BY INTERNATIONAL BODIES			162

1. SUMMARY AND EVALUATION, CONCLUSIONS AND RECOMMENDATIONS

1.1 Summary and evaluation

1.1.1 *Use, environmental fate, and environmental levels*

1,2-Dichloropropane is a liquid with a boiling point of 96.8 °C and a vapour pressure of 42 mmHg at 20 °C. The substance is soluble in water, ethanol, and ethyl ether. When heated, it emits highly toxic fumes of phosgene. The log P octanol/water partition coefficient is 2.28.

This substance is used in furniture finish, dry cleaning fluid, and paint remover, gum processing, metal degreasing, oil processing, and as a rubber- and wax-making agent, and a chemical intermediate in the production of tetrachloroethylene and carbon tetrachloride. It is a component of the "MIX D/D", used as a pre-plant fumigant.

Concentrations of 1,2-dichloropropane in city air have been measured at 1.2 $\mu g/m^3$ (mean value), 0.021-0.040 $\mu g/m^3$, and 0.0065-1.4 $\mu g/m^3$ in Philadelphia, Portland, and Japan, respectively. Decomposition in the atmosphere is slow; on the basis of reaction with hydroxyl radicals, the half-life of 1,2-dichloropropane was > 313 days. Phototransformation is likely to be the dominant process for the decomposition. Adsorption on to particulate matter is necessary for appreciable phototransformation. Volatilization is likely to be the major route of loss from water.

In soil, the main routes of loss are volatilization and diffusion. 1,2-dichloropropane is persistent in soil. More than 98% of the 1,2-dichloropropane applied to loam soil was recovered 12-20 weeks after treatment.

Leaching of 1,2-dichloropropane occurs from soil and can contaminate upper and lower groundwater in areas where "MIX D/D" has been used as a soil fumigant. In well water and groundwater in the USA, concentrations of up to 440 $\mu g/litre$ and 51 $\mu g/litre$, respectively, have been found. In the Netherlands, concentrations of up to 160 $\mu g/litre$ have been measured in well water and 1,2-dichloropropane has been found to a depth of 13 m.

1,2-Dichloropropane can be taken up by edible crops, but the residues detected have been low (< 0.01 mg/kg) and are unlikely to be biologically significant.

Bioaccumulation of 1,2-dichloropropane is unlikely, because of its high water solubility (2.7 g/kg) and low log P octanol/water partition coefficient.

1.1.2 Kinetics and metabolism

1,2-Dichloropropane administered orally to rats is rapidly eliminated (80-90% within 24 h). There are no major differences in kinetics or elimination between males and females. Urine is the major route of elimination, up to half an oral dose being eliminated by this route within 24 h. Less than 10% is eliminated via the faeces. Approximately one-third is eliminated through expired air, both as carbon dioxide and as a mixture of volatile materials. Tissue concentrations are low, the highest concentration being found in the liver. Rapid elimination also occurs following the inhalation exposure of rats; 55-65% of a dose is eliminated in the urine and 16-23% in expired air. The half-life of elimination from the blood is 24-30 min.

Unchanged 1,2-dichloropropane is not found in urine. Three major urinary metabolites have been identified. These metabolites result from oxidative and conjugation pathways, which yield the mercapturates, N-acetyl-S-(2-hydroxypropyl)-L-cysteine, N-acetyl-S-(2-oxypropyl)-L-cysteine, and N-acetyl-S-(1-carboxyethyl)-L-cysteine. 1,2-Dichloropropane can also be oxidized to lactate with resultant carbon dioxide or acetyl co-enzyme A production.

Oral administration of 1,2-dichloropropane (2 ml/kg) to rats significantly depleted tissue glutathione contents. There was a correlation between tissue glutathione loss and expression of toxicity in the liver, kidneys, and red blood cells. Prior depletion of intracellular glutathione exacerbated 1,2-dichloropropane toxicity, whereas pretreatment with precursors for glutathione synthesis ameliorated the toxicity. These results demonstrate the protective effect of glutathione against 1,2-dichloropropane toxicity.

1.1.3 Effects on organisms in the environment

EC_{50} for freshwater algae have not been calculated because of difficulties with volatilization of the chemical from the test solution. The acute toxicity of 1,2-dichloropropane for aquatic invertebrates and fish is low to moderate; 48-h LC_{50} values for invertebrates range between 52 and > 100 mg/litre and 96-h LC_{50} values for fish lie between 61 and 320 mg/litre. A short-term toxicity test on Fathead minnows demonstrated a maximum no-effect level of 82 mg/litre. A 32-day test on early life stage toxicity in the same species demonstrated that larval growth and survival were the most sensitive parameters. The estimated maximum acceptable toxicant concentration (MATC) was between 6 and 11 mg/litre. Growth inhibition was noted in Sheepshead minnows after 33 days at a 1,2-dichloropropane concentration of 164 mg/litre.

1,2-Dichloropropane is phytotoxic.

Contact tests on 4 species of earthworm showed an LC_{50} of 44-84 $\mu g/cm^2$ (mean values) of filter paper. In artificial soil, the LC_{50} values were 3880-5300 mg/kg soil (dry weight).

1.1.4 Effects on experimental animals and in vitro test systems

The acute oral toxicity of 1,2-dichloropropane in experimental animals is low. The oral LD_{50} for the rat is 1.9 g/kg body weight, and the dermal LD_{50} in rabbits is 8.75 ml/kg body weight.

Short-term, oral toxicity studies of 1,2-dichloropropane in mice and rats showed growth inhibition, clinical toxic signs associated with central nervous system depression, and/or increased mortality at dose levels of 250 mg/kg body weight per day or higher. In rats given 250 mg/kg per day for 10 days, there were changes in serum enzymes indicative of slight hepatotoxicity with a NOEL of 100 mg/kg per day.

In a 13-week mouse inhalation study (highest dose 681 mg/m^3), no adverse effects were observed. In a similar study on rats exposed to 68.1, 227, or 681 mg/m^3, a decrease in body weight and minimal damage to nasal tissues occurred in the 2 highest dose groups.

In a 2-generation reproduction study, rats exposed to 1,2-dichloropropane in drinking-water at 0.024, 0.1, 0.24% (equivalent to 33.6, 140 and 336 mg/kg body weight per day) resulted in lower maternal body weight gain and decreased water consumption at the mid and high dose levels. Neonatal body weights were lower at the high dose level. The NOAELs established for maternal and reproductive toxicity were 33.6 and 140 mg/kg body weight per day, respectively.

Studies did not indicate any teratogenic activity of 1,2-dichloropropane at oral dose levels up to 125 mg/kg body weight in the rat and 150 mg/kg body weight in the rabbit. However, at these dose levels, 1,2-dichloropropane was maternally toxic and fetotoxic, as evidenced by central nervous system associated clinical signs, decreased maternal body weight gain, and delayed ossification of bones in the fetuses. The NOELs are 30 and 50 mg/kg body weight per day for the rat and rabbit, respectively.

1,2-Dichloropropane was mutagenic in bacteria in most studies with, and without, metabolic activation, but very high dose levels were used of up to 10 mg/plate. In Chinese hamster ovary cells, 1,2-dichloropropane caused chromosomal aberrations and sister chromatid exchange; in Chinese hamster V79 cells, it increased the sister chromatid exchange. In an *in vitro* system with human lymphocytes, the tritiated thymidine uptake and cell viability in cultures grown with, and without, rat liver metabolizing system, were similar to those in control cultures. The results of a sex-linked recessive lethal test in *Drosophila melanogaster* were negative. A dominant lethal test in rats, dosed for 14 weeks via drinking-water containing 1,2-dichloropropane, followed by 2 weeks of mating, was negative.

In a carcinogenicity study on mice administered 125 or 250 mg 1,2-dichloropropane/kg body weight by gavage, a dose-related increase in the incidence of liver adenomas was observed. The incidence of liver adenomas in treated groups was higher than that in the concurrent control group, but was within the historical control range.

In rats administered dose levels of 125 and 250 mg/kg body weight (females) and 62 and 125 mg/kg body weight (males), by gavage, for 5 days per week over 113 weeks, a slight increase in the incidence of mammary gland adenocarcinomas exceeding the historical range was observed in high-dose females.

1.1.5 Effects on human beings

Exposure of the general population to 1,2-dichloropropane via air and water is unlikely, except in areas where there is extensive use of 1,2-dichloropropane and "MIX D/D" in agriculture. Residues of 1,2-dichloropropane in edible crops are generally below the limit of detection. In view of these low exposures to 1,2-dichloropropane, the risk to the general population is negligible.

Several cases of acute poisoning have been reported due to accidental or intentional (suicide) over-exposure to 1,2-dichloropropane. Effects have been mainly on the central nervous system, liver, and kidneys. Haemolytic anaemia and disseminated intravascular coagulation have also been reported. In one case, delirium progressed to irreversible shock, cardiac failure, and death.

Occupational exposures can be via both skin and inhalation. Several cases of dermatitis and skin sensitization have been reported in workers using solvent mixtures containing 1,2-dichloropropane.

1.2 Conclusions

- **General population**: There is low or non-existent exposure of the general population to 1,2-dichloropropane from air and food. However, in certain areas, exposure may occur when groundwater is contaminated.

- **Occupational exposure**: With good work practices, hygienic measures, and safety precautions, the use of 1,2-dichloropropane is unlikely to present a risk for those occupationally exposed to it.

- **Environment**: 1,2-Dichloropropane is unlikely to attain levels of environmental significance when used at the recommended rate. It is unlikely to have adverse effects on populations of terrestrial and aquatic organisms.

1.3 Recommendations

- Studies should be conducted to assess acute inhalation toxicity, eye and skin irritancy, and skin sensitization potential.

- Appropriate safety precautions should be taken, when handling 1,2-dichloropropane, in order to avoid exposures exceeding the maximum allowable concentration.

2. IDENTITY, PHYSICAL AND CHEMICAL PROPERTIES, ANALYTICAL METHODS

2.1 Identity

Primary constituent

Chemical structure

$$\mathrm{ClCH_2\underset{\underset{\displaystyle Cl}{|}}{C}HCH_3}$$

Chemical formula $C_3H_6Cl_2$

Relative molecular mass   112.99

Chemical name   1,2-dichloropropane, dichloro-1,2-propane

Common synonyms   propylene dichloride

CAS registry number   78-87-5

RTECS registry number   TX9625000

EINECS number   201-152-2

2.2 Physical and chemical properties

1,2-Dichloropropane is a liquid with a boiling point of 96.8 °C. The vapour pressure is 42 mmHg at 20 °C (27.9 kPa at 19.6 °C). Its solubility is 2.7 g/kg water at 20 °C. It is soluble in ethanol and diethyl ether. The density is 1.1595 g/ml at 20 °C, and 1.437 g/ml at 25 °C. It is flammable; the flash point is 21 °C (Cleveland open cup). When heated to decomposition, 1,2-dichloropropane emits highly toxic fumes of phosgene.

The log P octanol/water partition coefficient is 2.28 (NTP, 1983).

2.3 Conversion factors

1 ppm = 4.66 mg/m^3
1 mg/m^3 = 0.214 ppm

2.4 Analytical methods

The analytical methods used are the same as those used for 1,3-dichloropropene.

Boyd et al. (1981) developed a method to collect vapours of 1,2-dichloropropane from air with solid sorbents (petroleum charcoal) in tandem with a personal sampling pump; desorption of the sorbed compound in acetone/cyclohexane and analysis of the extracts by gas chromatography. A Carbowax or Chromosorb column was used. The Hall electrolytic conductivity detector (in the halogen mode) offered better sensitivity than the electron-capture detector and the flame ionization detector.

An analytical method is described and issued in 1985 by NIOSH, method 1013, for the determination of 1,2-dichloropropane in air. The working range is 0.25-600 mg/m^3. The limit of determination 0.1 µg/sample (NIOSH, 1985).

In method MDHS 28, a description is given for the determination of the time-weighted-average concentrations of chlorinated hydrocarbon solvent vapours in workplace atmospheres. The method is suitable for sampling over periods in the range of 10 min to 8 h. The method can also be used for the determination of personal exposure. The method is suitable for the measurement of airborne vapours containing concentrations in the range of approximately 1-1000 mg/m^3 (about 0.2-200 ppm v/v) for samples of 10 litres of air. Charcoal is used as adsorbent and 15% (v/v) acetone in cyclohexane is recommended as a desorption solvent for 1,2-dichloropropane; determination takes place with a gas chromatograph fitted with a flame ionization detector (HSE, 1990).

See section 2.4 of 1,3-dichloropropene.

3. SOURCES OF HUMAN AND ENVIRONMENTAL EXPOSURE

3.1 Natural occurrence

1,2-Dichloropropane is not known to occur naturally.

3.2 Man-made sources

1,2-Dichloropropane is produced by the chlorination of propylene.

The production of 1,2-dichloropropane in the USA in 1974 was 66 million kg: in 1976, it was 32.2 million, and in 1980, 35 million kg (Fishbein, 1979).

1,3-Dichloropropene, contaminated with 1,2-dichloropropane and 2,3-dichloropropene, used for fumigation in the Netherlands at application rates ranging from 200 to 400 kg/ha, would mean an input of 40-160 kg of 1,2-dichloropropane and 10-25 kg of 2,3-dichloropropenes/ha (Krijgsheld & van der Gen, 1986). 1,2-Dichloropropane is more persistent in the environment than 1,3-dichloropropene and has a greater potential for contaminating groundwater, because of its slow chemical degradation. By reducing the 1,2-dichloropropane content of the products used in agriculture, the contamination of groundwater will decrease.

3.3 Uses

1,2-Dichloropropane is a solvent for fats and oils. It has also been used as an insecticide fumigant on grain and soil and to control peach tree borers. Other uses are in gum processing, oil processing, and organic chemical synthesis, in rubber making, wax making, and the making of scouring compounds (Fishbein, 1979; Sittig, 1980; Baruffini et al., 1989). It is used in furniture finishing, dry cleaning fluid, paint remover, and metal degreasing, and is a chemical intermediate for the production of tetrachloroethylene and carbon tetrachloride (Fishbein, 1979).

It is a component of "MIX D/D" (Sittig, 1980; Worthing & Hance, 1991).

4. ENVIRONMENTAL TRANSPORT, DISTRIBUTION, AND TRANSFORMATION

4.1 Transport and distribution between media

4.1.1 Air

Phototransformation is likely to be the dominant process for the decomposition of 1,2-dichloropropane, but vapour phase photolysis was not detected after prolonged simulated sunlight irradiation in a reaction chamber (California State Water Resources Control Board, 1983).

Adsorption on to particulate matter seems to be necessary for appreciable direct phototransformation. The decomposition is rather slow in the atmosphere. It was calculated that, on the basis of reaction with hydroxyl radicals, the half-life of 1,2-dichloropropane was > 313 days for a 24-h average OH-radical concentration of 1×10^6 cm^3 (Tuazon et al., 1984).

See also section 4.1.1 of 1,3-dichloropropene.

4.1.2 Soil

The persistence of 1,3-dichloropropene and 1,2-dichloropropane depends on chemical transformation, volatilization, microbial transformation, photochemical transformation, and uptake into organisms (see section 4.1.3.5 and Table 5 on 1,3-dichloropropene and section 4.3.2 and Table 23 on "MIX D/D"). The persistence and degradation depend on the type of soil and the temperature (Sittig, 1980).

Little or no chemical degradation of 1,2-dichloropropane has been observed in laboratory and field studies. More than 98% of 1,2-dichloropropane applied to a sandy loam soil and medium loam soil was recovered 12-20 weeks after treatment (Roberts & Stoydin, 1976).

4.1.2.1 Volatilization

See section 4.1.3.2 of 1,3-dichloropropene.

4.1.2.2 Uptake in crops

See section 4.1.3.3 of 1,3-dichloropropene.

4.1.2.3 Movement in soil

See section 4.1.3.4 of 1,3-dichloropropene.

4.2 Biotransformation

In a well-run, waste-water treatment plant, Bi-Chem mutant bacteria can remove chlorinated aliphatic hydrocarbons, such as 1,2-dichloropropane (Straley et al., 1982).

Oldenhuis et al. (1989) studied the conversion of 1,2-dichloropropane by the methanotrophic bacterium *Methylosinus trichosporium* OB3b, grown in continuous cultures. 1,2-Dichloropropane was added at a concentration of 0.2 mmol/litre. After 24 h, complete degradation was found. 2,3-Dichloro-1-propanol was identified as a degradation product.

4.3 Bioconcentration

No data on bioconcentration are available.

5. ENVIRONMENTAL LEVELS AND HUMAN EXPOSURE

5.1 Environmental levels

5.1.1 Air

The City of Philadelphia made an emission inventory of 99 pollutants. In the periods 11 December 1983 to 31 March 1984 and 6 February 1984 to 31 March 1984, the mean concentration of 1,2-dichloropropane observed in the air was 1.2 $\mu g/m^3$ (Haemisegger et al., 1985; Sullivan et al., 1985).

In Portland, Oregon, the atmospheric gas-phase concentration of 1,2-dichloropropane during rain events in the period February-April 1984, ranged between 21 and 40 ng/m^3 (Ligocki et al., 1985).

In Japan, ambient air levels of 1,2-dichloropropane were monitored in 13 cities in 1989. The substance was detected in 11 out of 36 samples at levels ranging from 0.0065 to 1.4 $\mu g/m^3$ (Japan Environment Agency, 1991, letter from Sawamura, Ministry of Health and Welfare, Tokyo, Japan, to the IPCS).

5.1.2 Water and soil

It was reported from the USA that 1.4% of 945 wells contained a median level of 0.9 μg 1,2-dichloropropane/litre. In Maryland, 13 out of 36 wells contained 1,2-dichloropropane at levels ranging from 1 to 440 μg/litre. In California, 3 wells out of 64 were positive for 1,2-dichloropropane, in another study, 12 out of 95 wells were positive with levels ranging from 0.4 to 16 μg/litre. In the North Coast area, 18 out of 24 wells were positive, with 4 with levels above 10 μg/litre (California State Water Resources Control Board, 1983).

Hallberg (1989) also reported on the presence of 1,2-dichloropropane in groundwater in the USA; 1,2-dichloropropane was found in 7 States, with a maximum concentration of 51 μg/litre in Massachusetts. Connors et al. (1990) found levels of 0.7-19.0 μg 1,2-dichloropropane/litre in potable water samples collected in 8 homes in 3 communities in Connecticut.

In 1984, micropollutants were analysed in well water in the northern part of the Netherlands in an area in which "MIX D/D" had been used for at least 20 years. 1,2-Dichloropropane was present in 14 out of 26 wells at levels ranging from 0.1 up to 9.2 µg/litre water (Hoogsteen, 1986).

Van Beek et al. (1988) studied the presence of 1,2-dichloropropane in well water in Noordbargeres in the potato growing area in the Northern Netherlands. Thirty-three wells were monitored and levels higher than 0.1 µg/litre were found in 17/45 samples. The highest concentration observed was 160 µg/litre. The 1,2-dichloropropane was found in well water up to a depth of 13 m. The average concentration of 1,2-dichloropropane (16 samples) found in Puttenveld in the northern Netherlands in a potato growing area, in the period 1985-86, was 1.1 µg/litre (range < 0.05-21.0 µg/litre) (Beugelink, 1987).

In 1987-88, samples of surface water up to 1 m depth were taken monthly at 5 sites in a polder in the Netherlands and analysed. The area is situated next to the dunes (where groundwater is being pumped up for the preparation of drinking-water) and is extensively used for bulb culture. The maximum concentration of 1,2-dichloropropane found was 16.2 µg/litre (Greve et al., 1989).

Lagas et al. (1989) analysed groundwater in 5 areas where potato, maize, and bulb crops were grown in the Netherlands. 1,2-Dichloropropane was found in 15 out of 22 samples of water collected to a depth of 6 m below potato crops in concentrations of < 0.1-200 µg/litre and in 6 out of 8 samples below maize and bulb crops in concentrations of < 1-14 µg/litre.

Cotruvo (1985) reported the occurrence of 1,2-dichloropropane in 6 out of 466 samples of groundwater (source not specified) in the USA. The median and maximum concentrations were 0.9 µg/litre and 21 µg/litre, respectively.

In Japan, 1,2-dichloropropane levels in water and bottom sediment were monitored at 26 points (7 mouth of river, 4 lake, 8 port and 7 bay areas) in 1989. The substance was detected in 20 out of 78 water samples with levels ranging from 0.00001 to 0.14 µg/litre and in 9 out of 78 sediment samples with levels ranging from 0.16 to 10.0 µg/kg (Japan Environment Agency, 1991, letter from Sawamura, Ministry of Health and Welfare, Tokyo, Japan, to the IPCS).

5.1.3 Crops

Residues of 1,2-dichloropropane in edible crop commodities, arising from the use of 1,3-dichloropropene or "MIX D/D", are generally below the limit of detection. The obvious reason for this, is that crops are not normally planted until most of the product applied has been dissipated. Another reason is that any 1,2-dichloropropane taken up by the plant, would have to survive the whole crop cycle to be detected in the harvested commodity.

Supervised trials with "MIX D/D", in 23 crops in 8 countries showed that residues in edible crop commodities were below the limits of determination (< 0.01 mg/kg), for 1,3-dichloropropene, 1,2-dichloropropane, and 3-chloroallyl alcohol.

6. KINETICS AND METABOLISM

6.1 Absorption, distribution, and elimination

6.1.1 Oral

Adult male and female Carworth Farm E rats received 1,2-dichloro[1-^{14}C]propane in 0.5 ml arachis oil, by stomach tube, and excretion was followed. After 4 days, the animals were killed and the radioactivity measured in the skin and carcass. The 24-h excretion of radioactivity was very rapid, 80-90% was eliminated in the faeces, urine, and expired air. The urine, the major route of excretion, contained 50.2% (average of male and female animals) of the administered dose. In expired air, 19.3% was found as labelled CO_2 and 23.1% as other volatile radioactivity. Only 4.4% was detected in the faeces in first 24 h. The skin and carcass contained 1.5 and 3.7% of the dose, respectively, on day 4 (Hutson et al., 1971).

In Sprague-Dawley rats, dosed orally with 20 mg 1,2-dichloropropane/kg body weight per day for 4 consecutive days, unchanged 1,2-dichloropropane was found in expired air, but not in the urine (Jones & Gibson, 1980).

^{14}C-1,2-Dichloropropane (99.9%) was administered orally to groups of 4 Fischer 344 rats/sex in a single dose of 1 or 100 mg/kg body weight, followed by 1 mg/kg per day non-radiolabelled compound for 7 days, and a single 1 mg dose of ^{14}C-1,2-dichloropropane/kg body weight on day 8. ^{14}C-1,2-Dichloropropane was rapidly absorbed, metabolized, and excreted in both sexes. In all treated groups, the principal routes of elimination were via the urine (37-52%), expired air (31-36%) and faeces (5.5-7.9%); a total of 80-90% was eliminated in the first 24 h. The tissues and carcass contained 7.1-10.6% of the dose. In general, the radioactivity was well distributed among the 13 organs and tissues analysed, 48 h after treatment. The liver contained the highest ^{14}C-activity in all groups; from 0.229 to 0.416% of the dose/g wet weight. Peak concentrations were found in the blood 4 h after treatment. The quantities of volatile organic compounds found ranged from 0.14 to 1.13% in the 1 mg/kg group and from 10 to 16% in the 100 mg/kg group; approximately 82% of the exhaled volatile organic compounds were in the form of 1,2-dichloropropane. Multiple exposure resulted in a statistically significant reduction in the amount of radioactivity eliminated in the urine, while the metabolism of 1,2-dichloropropane to CO_2 was enhanced. At 100 mg/kg, there was a significant reduction of CO_2 formation and enhancement of ^{14}C elimination as volatile organic compounds (14.7-33.4%) compared with a single dose. No parent 1,2-dichloropropane was found in the urine, but 3 mercapturic acid metabolites of 1,2-dichloropropane were identified (Timchalk et al., 1989).

6.1.2 Inhalation

Groups of 4 Fischer 344 rats/sex were exposed to ^{14}C-1,2-dichloropropane vapour for a 6-h period in head-only inhalation chambers at target concentrations of 23.3, 233, or 466 mg/m^3. The ^{14}C-1,2-dichloropropane was rapidly absorbed, metabolized, and excreted. The urine contained between 55 and 65% of the dose, and expired air contained 16-23% of $^{14}CO_2$. With increasing dose, a greater percentage of the recovered dose was eliminated as expired organic volatile compounds, i.e., 1.7, 2.1-3.4, and 6.3-6.7%, respectively. At 466 mg/m^3, this increase was statistically significant. The faeces contained 6.3-9.7% of the dose and the tissues and carcass accounted for 5.8-10.0%. No sex difference was noted. Radioactivity was well distributed among all 13 organs when the tissues were analysed after 48 h. The liver and kidneys had the highest concentration ranging from 0.154 to 0.292% and from 0.098 to 0.252% of the dose/g wet weight, respectively. Peak blood concentrations of 0.06, 0.92, and 3.87 µg/g blood for the 3 dose levels, respectively, were found at 4 h. Half-lives for elimination from blood were 24 and 30 min for females and males, respectively. No parent 1.2-dichloropropane was found in the urine, but 3 mercapturic acid metabolites were identified (section 6.2) (Timchalk et al., 1989).

6.1.3 Intraperitoneal

Groups of 5 male Wistar rats (200 g) were administered, i.p., 0, 10, 25, 50, 100, 250, or 500 mg 1,2-dichloropropane (97%)/kg body weight in 0.5 ml corn oil for 5 days (once daily) or for 4 weeks (five days/week). Urinary mercapturic acid excretion was monitored. A significant increase in mercapturic acid excretion was observed at all dose levels, with no further increase during the treatment: at lower doses, a return to baseline values occurred within 48 h of the end of the treatment. Mercapturic acid excretion at the end of weeks 2, 3, and 4 was significantly lower than that observed at the end of the first week (Trevisan et al., 1989).

6.2 Metabolic transformation

1,2-Dichloropropane is metabolized to form a variety of metabolic products. Dichloropropane oxidation yielded the mercapturic acid, N-acetyl-S-(2-hydroxypropyl)cysteine (Jones & Gibson, 1980). Three mercapturic acid metabolites were identified in the urine of Fischer 344 rats (110-140 g) administered 1,2-dichloropropane orally (100 mg/kg body weight) or by inhalation (466 mg/m^3 per 6 h). These compounds are N-acetyl-S-(2-hydroxypropyl)-L-cysteine, N-acetyl-S-(2-oxopropyl)-L-cysteine and N-acetyl-S-(1-carboxyethyl)-L-cysteine. Fischer 344 rats were given a single oral dose of deuterium (D6)-labelled dichloropropane (105 mg/kg body weight) in a mechanistic study conducted to determine whether the conjugated metabolites are generated through a sulfonium ion intermediate. The results suggest that dichloropropane undergoes oxidation either prior to, or subsequent to, glutathione conjugation. There was no evidence to support the existence of a sulfonium intermediate in the formation of the 2-hydroxypropyl-mercapturic acid metabolite of dichloropropane (Fig. 8). Instead, this metabolite is thought to arise via the direct oxidation of 1,2-dichloropropane, either prior to, or following, conjugation with glutathione (Fig. 8) (Timchalk et al., 1989; Bartels & Timchalk, 1990).

Imberti et al. (1990) investigated the effects of a single dose of 1,2-dichloropropane of 2 ml/kg body weight (by gavage) on the intracellular glutathione (GSH) content of the liver, kidneys, and blood of male Wistar rats (180-250 g). 1,2-Dichloropropane, administered orally, caused a significant depletion of GSH within 24 h of treatment, followed by a slow recovery, approaching normal levels after 96 h. The GSH depletion was associated with a marked increase in serum GOT, GPT, 5'-nucleotidase, gamma-glutamyl transpeptidase, alkaline phosphatase, urea, and creatinine, and a significant degree of haemolysis. The administration of L-buthionine-S,R sulfoximine (BSO) (0.5 g/kg body weight, i.p.), 4 h before 1,2-dichloropropane treatment, resulted in a significant increase in overall mortality. The administration of a GSH precursor, N-acetylcysteine (NAC), i.p., at 250 mg/kg body weight, 2 and 16 h after 1,2-dichloropropane treatment, prevented the loss of cellular GSH and reduced the extent of injury in the target tissues. There was a correlation between the depletion of liver GSH and the increases in GOT, GPT, and 5'-nucleotidase, between the depletion of GSH in the kidneys and the increase in serum urea and creatinine, and the depletion of GSH in blood and the occurrence of haemolysis.

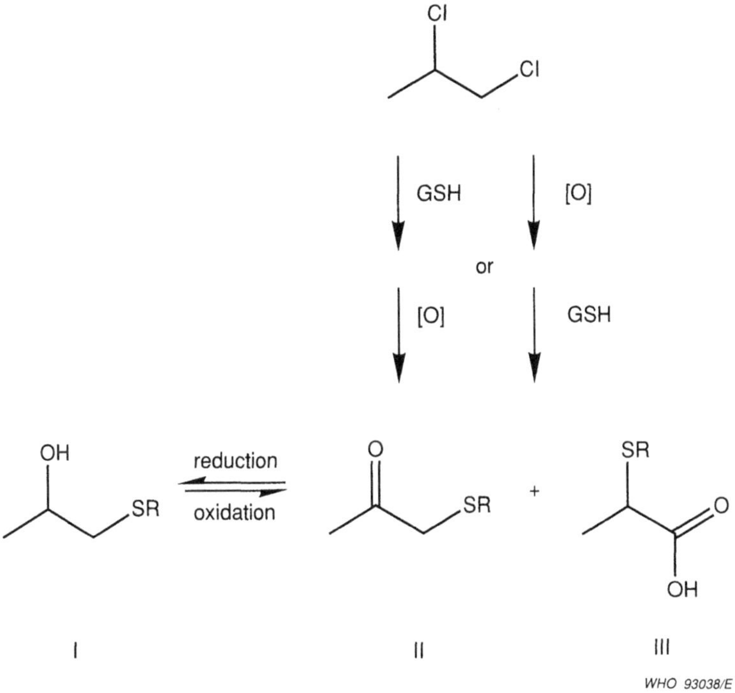

Fig. 8. Proposed metabolic scheme for the formation of mercapturic acid metabolites of 1,2-dichloropropane in the rat.
I   = N-acetyl-S-(2-hydroxypropyl)-L-cysteine;
II   = N-acetyl-S-(2-oxopropyl)-L-cysteine;
III = N-acetyl-S-(1-carboxyethyl)-L-cysteine.
Adapted from: Bartels & Timchalk (1990).

Both 1-chloro-2-hydroxypropane (II) and 1,2-epoxypropane (III) are proposed as intermediates in the metabolism to the mercapturic acid. 1,2-Epoxypropane can also be metabolized to propanediol (IV), which is further metabolized to pyruvate and enters the tricarboxylic acid cycle; carbon dioxide is released and expired. Epoxypropane may also be conjugated with glutathione (VI) and excreted in the urine. Jones & Gibson (1980) further proposed that the 1-chloro-2-hydroxypropane (II) may be metabolized to beta-chlorolactaldehyde (VII) and beta-chlorolactate (VIII) (Fig. 9).

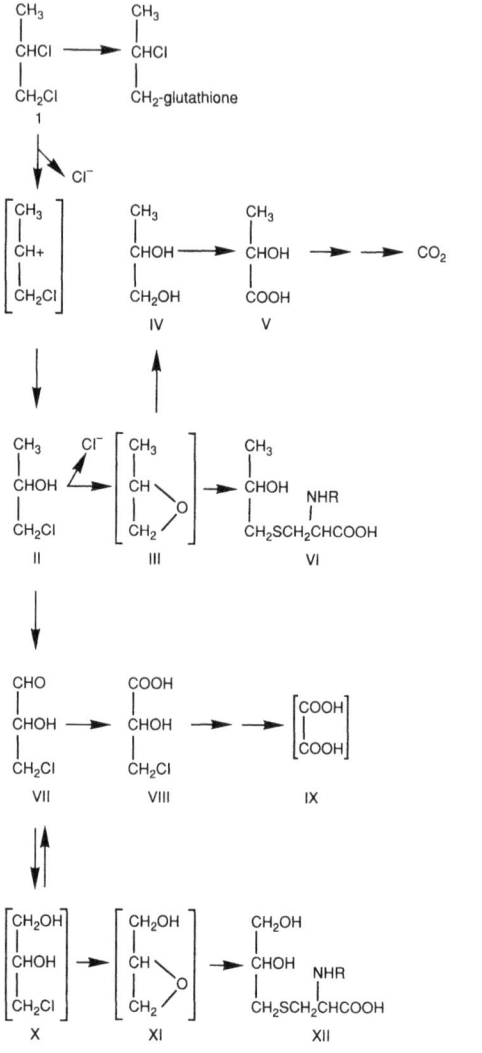

Fig. 9. The proposed metabolic pathways of 1,2-dichloropropane in the rat. Compounds in parentheses are proposed intermediates.
From: Jones & Gibson (1980).

7. EFFECTS ON ORGANISMS IN THE ENVIRONMENT

7.1 Aquatic organisms

7.1.1 Algae

The EC_{50} for CO_2 uptake by marine algae (*Phaeodactylum tricornutum*) was 50 mg/litre. 1,2-Dichloropropane was not found to exhibit any algistatic or algicidal effects in an acute toxicity study on *Selenastrum capricornutum*, though the problems of losses of 1,2-dichloropropane from the test flasks, made it impossible to calculate EC values (Dynamic Corporation, 1991).

A general trend of decreasing algal population growth with increasing nominal concentrations of 1,2-dichloropropane was observed in an acute toxicity test on *Skeletonema costatum*. Because the concentrations measured for each nominal value were variable, it was not appropriate to determine EC values. A NOEL of 18 mg/litre was determined, though it was not possible to distinguish algistatic from algicidal effects (Dynamic Corporation, 1991).

7.1.2 Invertebrates

The acute toxicity of 1,2-dichloropropane for non-target invertebrates is summarized in Table 18; 1,2-dichloropropane has a 48-h LC_{50} of 50-100 mg/litre for these aquatic organisms. No discernible effects on *Daphnia magna* were found at concentrations of less than 22 mg/litre (Leblanc, 1980).

Table 18. Acute toxicity of 1,2-dichloropropane in non-target aquatic insects and crustacea

Species	Temperature (°C)	48-h LC_{50} mg/litre	References
Barnacle nauplii (*Elminius moderatus*)	-	53	Pearson & McConnell (1975)
Brown shrimp (*Crangon crangon*)	-	> 100	Portmann & Wilson (1971)

7.1.3 Fish

7.1.3.1 Acute toxicity

The 96-h LC_{50} of 1,2-dichloropropane for freshwater and marine fish is 61-320 mg/litre (Table 19).

7.1.3.2 Short-term/long-term toxicity

Two embryo-larval tests have been conducted on Fathead minnow (*Pimephales promelas*) exposed to 1,2-dichloropropane. The maximum no-effect levels were 8.1 and 60 mg/litre, respectively (US EPA, 1980).

In the marine environment, growth inhibition was noted in the Sheepshead minnow (*Cyprinodon variegatus*) after 33 days exposure to 164 mg 1,2-dichloropropane/litre (US EPA, 1980).

A 32-day test to study early life stage toxicity in Fathead minnows (*Pimephales promelas*) demonstrated that larval growth and survival (28-day-old fish) were the most sensitive indicators of toxic effects. Embryo hatch and larval deformities at hatch were the least sensitive indicators of toxicity. The 1,2-dichloropropane (98%) was tested at dose levels of 0, 6, 11, 25, 51, and 110 mg/litre (temperature of the water 25 °C, hardness 45 mg/litre as $CaCO_3$, pH 7.4). The estimated maximum acceptable toxicant concentration (MATC) was between 6 and 11 mg/litre (Benoit et al., 1982).

7.2 Terrestrial organisms

7.2.1 Earthworms

Neuhauser et al. (1985a,b; 1986) studied the toxicity of 1,2-dichloropropane for 4 species of earthworm (*Allolobophora tuberculata, Eisenia foetida, Eudrilus eugeniae* and *Perionyx excavatus*) using EEC earthworm artificial soil and a contact testing procedure (Edwards, 1983). The LC_{50} values and 95% confidence limits in the contact test were 84(65-110); 64(59-70); 44(38-51); and 63(56-72) µg/cm² of filter paper for the 4 species of earthworms, respectively. In the artificial soil test, the LC_{50} values were 4272, 4240, 5300, and 3880 mg/kg dry weight artificial soil, respectively.

7.2.2 Plants

1,2-Dichloropropane is highly phytotoxic.

Table 19. Acute toxicity of 1,2-dichloropropane in fish

Species	Size or age	Temperature (°C)	96-h LC_{50} mg/litre	References
Guppy (*Poecilia reticulata*)	2-3 months	21-23	3.01 μmol/litre[f]	Könemann (1981)
Bluegill sunfish (*Lepomis macrochirus*)	33-75 mm 0.32-1.2 g	23[a] 21-23	320 280[b,c] (220-340)	Dawson et al. (1977) Buccafusco et al. (1981)
Fathead minnow (*Pimephales promelas*)	30-35 days	25[d,e]	140[d] (131-150)	Wallbridge (1983)
Tidewater silversides (*Menida beryllina*)	40-100 mm	20[a]	240	Dawson et al. (1977)
Dab (*Pleuronectes limanda*)	15-20 cm	-	61	Pearson & McConnell (1975)

[a] Hardness 55 mg/litre (as $CaCO_3$), pH 7.6-7.9.
[b] Tested in well-water, 32-48 mg/litre $CaCO_3$, pH 6.5-7.9, oxygen concentration at the beginning 9.7 to 0.3 mg/litre after 96-h exposure.
[c] Static system (nominal concentrations).
[d] Flow-through system.
[e] Hardness 42-45 mg/litre (as $CaCO_3$) pH 6.7-7.6.
[f] 7-day LC_{50} (static system, renewal).

8. EFFECTS ON EXPERIMENTAL ANIMALS AND *IN VITRO* TEST SYSTEMS

8.1 Single exposures

The acute oral LD_{50} for the rat has been reported to be 1.9 (1.7-2.1) g/kg body weight and the dermal LD_{50} after a single skin exposure of rabbits was 8.75 (8.3-9.2) ml/kg body weight (Smyth et al., 1969; California State Water Resources Control Board, 1983).

8.2 Short-term exposures

8.2.1 Oral

8.2.1.1 Mouse

Groups of 5 male and 5 female $B_6C_3F_1$ mice were administered (by gavage) 0, 125, 250, 500, 1000, or 2000 mg 1,2-dichloropropane (99.4%) per kg body weight, in corn oil. The doses were given for 14 consecutive days (range-finding study) followed by 1 day of observation. All male mice in the 1000 and 2000 mg/kg groups and female mice in the 2000 mg/kg group died. Also 3 out of 5 males receiving 500 mg/kg and 4 out of 5 females receiving 1000 mg/kg died. No growth inhibition was seen in the surviving animals (NTP, 1986).

Groups of 10 male and 10 female $B_6C_3F_1$ mice were then administered 1,2-dichloropropane (99.4%) in corn oil, by gavage, 5 days per week for 13 weeks, at doses of 0, 30, 60, 125, 250, or 500 mg/kg body weight. Mortality was not significantly increased, and mean body weight changes were not dose-related. No compound-related histopathological changes were found at the highest dose level (NTP, 1986).

8.2.1.2 Rat

Groups of 5 male and 5 female F344/N rats were administered 1,2-dichloropropane (99.4%) at 0, 125, 250, 500, 1000, and 2000 mg/kg body weight, in corn oil, by gavage, for 14 consecutive days (range-finding study) followed by 1 day of observation. All rats receiving the highest dose level died. Growth inhibition was seen in the surviving animals in the 1000 mg/kg group. At necropsy, renal medullae were red in the 2000 mg/kg group, not in lower dose levels (NTP, 1986).

Groups of 10 male and 10 female F344/N rats were then administered 1,2-dichloropropane (99.4%) in corn oil, by gavage, 5 days per week for 13 weeks at doses of 0, 60, 125, 250, 500, or 1000 mg/kg body weight. All animals administered 1000 mg/kg and half of the males administered 500 mg/kg died. Growth inhibition was seen in the 500 mg/kg group. Centrilobular congestion of the liver occurred in the 1000 mg/kg group and 2 females of this group showed hepatic changes and centrilobular necrosis. Lower dose levels did not produce effects (NTP, 1986).

A 2-week study of 1,2-dichloropropane (99.9%) was conducted using groups of 10 Fischer 344 rats/sex to select doses for a subsequent 13-week study. Dose levels were 0 (corn oil), 300, or 500 mg/kg body weight per day (by gavage) for 14 days. Data were obtained on body weight, clinical effects, body temperature, functional observational battery, motor activity, haematology, liver, kidney, and spleen weights, gross pathology and histological examination of the liver and kidneys. In both groups, transient clinical effects (tearing, blinking, and lethargy) were seen, and body weights were significantly decreased. The body temperatures of treated animals in both groups, recorded 1 h after dosing on day 13, were decreased by 0.3-0.5 °C. No effects on motor activity and haematology were noted. Liver and kidney weights were increased and spleen weight decreased. Histopathological changes (prominent nucleoli of hepatocytes in the centrilobular region, degeneration and necrosis of the liver cells) were found in the livers of animals in both the treated groups (Gorzinski & Johnson, 1989).

In an oral toxicity study, adult male Sprague-Dawley rats were administered 0, 100, 250, 500, or 1000 mg 1,2-dichloropropane/kg body weight, in corn oil (by gavage), once a day, for up to 10 consecutive days. Some rats were killed at each dose level 24 h after 1, 5, and 10 daily doses. After dosing, changes in body weight and clinical toxic signs were assessed. In addition, measurements of clinical chemistry parameters, urinary levels of glucose, alkaline and acid phosphatase and N-acetyl glycosaminidase activities, and the histopathology of major organs, liver enzyme levels, as well as levels of non-protein sulfhydryls in the liver and kidneys were determined. Definite central nervous system depression and body weight loss, and increased renal nonprotein sulfhydryl (NPS) levels were seen at 250 mg/kg. Liver damage (both morphological and enzyme changes) was observed only at the 500 and 1000 mg/kg dose levels. In this study, "resistance" to 1,2-dichloropropane hepatotoxicity developed over the 10 consecutive days of exposure, as reflected by progressively lower serum enzyme levels and by decreases in the severity and incidence of toxic hepatitis and periportal vacuolization. Nucleolar enlargement in hepatocytes, however, was observed at all dose levels at both 5 and 10 days. There were a number of manifestations of haemolytic anaemia in various tissues, but no evidence of nephrotoxicity. On the basis of the parameters examined, a NOEL of 100 mg/kg body weight can be established (Bruckner et al., 1989).

In a similar oral study, male Sprague-Dawley adult rats were treated with 0, 100, 250, 500, or 750 mg 1,2-dichloropropane/kg body weight, in corn oil, by gavage, 5 times weekly for up to 13 weeks. Over one-half of the animals in the 750 mg/kg group died within 10 days. Histopathological changes included mild hepatitis and splenic haemosiderosis, adrenal medullary vacuolization and cortical lipidosis, testicular degeneration and a reduction in sperm, and an increased number of degenerated spermatogonia in the epididymis. Similar testicular and epididymal degenerative changes were observed in some animals in the 500 mg/kg group after 13 weeks of dosing. While no deaths occurred in the 100 or 250 mg/kg groups, more than 50% in the 500 mg/kg group had died by 13 weeks. A dose-dependent decrease in body weight gain was observed. 1,2-Dichloropropane exhibited very limited hepatotoxic potential and no apparent nephrotoxic potential in this 13-week study (Bruckner et al., 1989).

8.2.2 Inhalation

8.2.2.1 Mouse

$B_6C_3F_1$ mice (aged 6-8 weeks) were exposed to target concentrations of 1,2-dichloropropane (99.9%) of 0, 69.9, 233, or 699 mg/m^3 for 6 h/day, 5 days/week, for 13 weeks. The mean actual concentrations were 0, 74.5, 233, or 694 mg/m^3. There were no effects on haematology, gross pathology, and histopathology at concentrations as high as 699 mg/m^3, in this study (Nitschke et al., 1988).

8.2.2.2 Rat

Fischer 344 rats (aged 6-8 weeks) were exposed to target concentrations of 0, 69.9, 233, or 699 mg 1,2-dichloropropane (99.9%)/m^3 for 6 h/day, 5 days/week, for 13 weeks. The mean actual concentrations were 0, 74.5, 233, or 694 mg/m^3. The body weights of rats exposed to 233 and 699 mg/m^3 were significantly decreased. Minimal effects were observed microscopically in the nasal tissues of rats exposed to 233 and 699 mg/m^3. A few rats exposed to 69.9 mg/m^3 also had slight thickening of a small portion of the respiratory nasal mucosa. No treatment-related effects were noted in haematology, clinical chemistry, or urinalysis, even at 699 mg/m^3 (Nitschke et al., 1988). A NOEL of 74.5 mg/m^3 can be established.

8.2.2.3 Rabbit

New Zealand white rabbits (age 6-7 months) were exposed to 1,2-dichloropropane at 0, 699, 2330, or 4660 mg/m^3 for 6 h/day, 5 days/week, for 13 weeks. The mean actual concentrations were 0, 694, 2204, or 4436 mg/m^3. Minimal effects on nasal tissues were present in male rabbits only at the 4660 mg/m^3 level. The primary effects, decreased red blood cell parameters (red cell blood count, haemoglobin, and packed cell volume), were observed in male rabbits exposed to 699 (minimal effects) - 4660 mg/m^3, and in female rabbits exposed to 2330 and 4660 mg/m^3 (Nitschke et al., 1988). No NOEL has been established.

8.3 Reproduction, embryotoxicity, and teratogenicity

8.3.1 Reproduction

Groups of 30 male and 30 female Sprague-Dawley rats each were provided with drinking-water containing 1,2-dichloropropane (99.9%) at concentrations of 0, 0.24, 1, or 2.4 g/litre (w/v) (equivalent to 0, 33.6, 140, or 336 mg/kg body weight) over 2 generations. A concentration of 2.4 g/litre represented the maximum practicable attainable concentration, based on solubility. Adult rats were evaluated for body weights, water and feed consumption, reproductive performance, and gross pathological and histological changes. The litters were evaluated for size, neonatal growth, and survival. Decreases in water consumption reflective of rejection because of unpalatability, were observed at all levels tested in both sexes in the F_0 and F_1 generations. These decreases in water consumption resulted in significantly lower body weights in both generations administered 2.4 g/litre. These differences in water consumption and body weights were also evident among the females during gestation and/or lactation. The 0.24 g/litre dose level had a minor effect on water consumption and body weights, but no adverse effects on the animals. No treatment-related gross pathological changes were noted in any dose group and the histological changes were limited to increased hepatocellular granularity in both sexes in both generations at all dose levels.

There were no histological changes in the reproductive tracts of either sex in either generation. Reproductive function, measured by fertility and litter size, was unaffected. The decreases in water consumption among females at 2.4 g 1,2-dichloropropane/litre resulted in significantly lower neonatal body weights and slightly increased neonatal mortality in their litters. These neonatal effects were considered secondary to the substantial decreases in maternal water consumption, rather than a direct effect of the substance. There were no neonatal effects at the 2 lower concentrations. The NOAEL for adults is 0.24 g/litre, and the reproductive NOAEL is 1 g/litre (equivalent to 140 mg/kg body weight) (Kirk et al., 1990).

8.3.2 Teratogenicity

8.3.2.1 Oral (rat)

Groups of 30 Sprague-Dawley rats were administered 1,2-dichloropropane (99.9%) in corn oil, by gavage, on gestation days 6-15 at dose levels of 0, 10, 30, or 125 mg/kg body weight per day. Parameters evaluated included maternal body weight and weight gain, feed and water consumption, fetal weights, and fetal morphology. The highest dose level produced transient decreases in respiration, movement, muscle tone and extensor thrust reflex, and increases in salivation and lacrimation, within 1 h of dosing on day 6 of gestation. A decrease in the frequency of these clinical symptoms occurred on the second day. In rats, 1,2-dichloropropane produced transient central nervous system depression and decreased maternal body weight gain and feed consumption at 125 mg/kg body weight. Fetal effects in rats were limited to a significant increase in the incidence of delayed ossification of the bones of the skull in the 125 mg/kg group, secondary to maternal effects. A level of 30 mg/kg was considered the NOEL for maternal and fetal effects (Kirk et al., 1989; Hanley et al., 1990).

8.3.2.2 Oral (rabbit)

Groups of 18 New Zealand white rabbits were administered 1,2-dichloropropane (99.9%) at dose levels of 0, 15, 50, or 150 mg/kg body weight per day on gestation days 7-19. On day 28 of gestation, Caesarean section was performed and the fetuses evaluated. Parameters evaluated included maternal body weight and weight gain, haematology, fetal body weights, and fetal morphology. In maternal rabbits, a dose of 150 mg/kg per day produced anorexia, significant decreases in weight gain, and anaemia, with microscopic examination revealing slight to moderate anisocytosis, poikilocytosis, and/or polychromasia, indicative of a regenerative anaemia. The only fetal effect in rabbits was a significant increase in the incidence of delayed ossification of the bones of the skull at the highest dose level, secondary to maternal effects. No effects were observed in the 15 and 50 mg/kg dose groups. The NOEL for both maternal and fetal effects was 50 mg/kg body weight (Hanley et al., 1989a).

8.4 Mutagenicity and related end-points

8.4.1 In vitro studies

8.4.1.1 Microorganisms

1,2-Dichloropropane was tested for its mutagenic activity in *Salmonella typhimurium*, *Saccharomyces cerevisiae* with, and without metabolic activation, and in *Aspergillus nidulans* and *Streptomyces coelicolor*. Results in most studies on *S. typhimurium* TA100 and TA1535 were positive, but negative results were obtained with TA98, TA1537, and TA1538, *S. cerevisiae*, and *S. coelicolor*. In *Aspergillus nidulans*, a forward mutation to 8-azaguanine resistance and methionine suppression was found with S9 activation.

The results are summarized in Table 20.

Crebelli et al. (1984) studied the induction of somatic segregation in *Aspergillus nidulans*. Induction of haploidization, mitotic non-disjunction, and mitotic crossing-over was studied in heterozygous colonies exposed to 1,2-dichloropropane, 99%. No significant rise in frequency of any kind of segregated sectors was found. The concentration that was used was 154 mmol/litre.

8.4.1.2 Mammalian cells

In cytogenetic studies using Chinese hamster ovary cells, 1,2-dichloropropane (99.4%) caused both chromosome aberrations and sister chromatid exchanges. Dose levels tested were 0.46-1.50 and 0.113-1.13 mg/ml, respectively (Galloway et al., 1987).

Table 20. Mutagenicity tests with 1,2-dichloropropane on microorganisms

Organism/strain	Substance	Dose	Type of test	Metabolic activation	Result	Reference
Salmonella typhimurium						
TA100, TA1535	1,2-DCP	10-50 mg	plate	S9 mix/none	+	De Lorenzo et al. (1977)
TA1978				S9 mix/none	-	
TA100	1,2-DCP (65%	62.5-8000	suspension	S9 mix	+	Priston et al. (1983)
TA1535	1,2-DCP + 25%	µg/ml^d		S9 mix/none	+	
	1,3-DCPropene)					
TA98, TA1537				S9 mix/none	-	
TA100	1,2-DCP	1, 10, 100 µmol^e	plate	S9 mix/none	-	Stolzenberg & Hine (1980)
TA100, TA1535	1,2-DCP	1-10 µlitre	plate	S9 mix/none	+	Carere & Morpurgo (1981)
TA98, TA1537, TA1538				S9 mix/none	-	
TA100, TA1535	1,2-DCP	0.33-10 mg	plate	S9 mix/none (rat/hamster)	+	Haworth et al. (1983)
TA98, TA1537				S9 mix/none (rat/hamster)	-	
TA100, TA1535, TA1537	1,2-DCP (99%)	33-2000 µg	plate	S9 mix	-	NTP (1983)
				S9 none	(+)	
TA98				S9 mix/none (rat/hamster)	-	

Table 20 (contd).

Organism/strain	Substance	Dose	Type of test	Metabolic activation	Result	Reference
Saccharomyces cerevisiae						
JD1	1,2-DCP (65%) 1,2-DCP + 25% 1,3-DC propene)	62.5-8000 µg/ml[d]	-	S9 mix S9 none	- (+)	Priston et al. (1983)
Streptomyces coelicolar[b] A3	1,2-DCP	2-100 µlitre	plate	none	-	Carere & Morpurgo (1981)
Aspergillus nidulans[c]		100-400 µlitre	plate	none	+	Carere & Morpurgo (1981)
Aspergillus nidulans	1,2-DCP (99%)	154 mmol/litre			-	Crebelli et al. (1984)

[a] The highest dose level, 100 µmol/plate gave complete inhibition of bacterial growth.
[b] Resistance to streptomycin.
[c] Resistance to 8-azaguanine.
[d] Concentrations of 1000 µg/ml and higher were cytotoxic.

Priston et al. (1983) also studied the ability of 1,2-dichloropropane (containing 65% 1,2-dichloropropane and 25% 1,3-dichloropropane) to induce chromosome damage using rat liver (RL_4) cells, in concentrations of 5-20 µg/ml. An indication for a small increase in the frequency of chromatid gaps, chromatid and chromosome aberrations, was noticed, but only in the presence of cytotoxic effects. The Task Group considered this study inadequate.

Von der Hude et al. (1987) used the Sister Chromatid Exchange test *in vitro* in Chinese hamster V79 cells to evaluate the effect of 1,2-dichloropropane (99%). The concentrations tested were 0 (DMSO), 1.0, 3.3, and 10.0 mmol/litre without S9 mix. A dose-related increase in SCEs was observed. With S9 mix and the same concentrations, the SCEs frequency was increased but was less than without S9 mix.

8.4.2 In vivo studies

8.4.2.1 Drosophila melanogaster

Woodruff et al. (1985) tested 1,2-dichloropropane at 0 and 4200 mg/litre by injection in germ cells and 0 and 33 552 mg/m³ by inhalation in *Drosophila melanogaster*, using the sex-linked recessive lethal mutation for their mutagenicity. The results by injection and inhalation were negative.

8.4.2.2 Dominant lethal test

Groups of 30 male Sprague-Dawley rats were given 1,2-dichloropropane (99.9%) in the drinking-water at concentrations of 0, 0.24, 1, or 2.4 g/litre, continuously, for a period of approximately 14 weeks, as part of a combined reproduction/dominant lethal study (section 8.3.1). Exposed males (F_0) were used for a dominant lethal test following completion of the breeding for the F_1 litters of the reproduction study. They were mated with pairs of naive, untreated adult females for 2 successive periods of 1 week each. A separate, positive control group of 30 male rats was administered a single oral dose of 100 mg cyclophosphamide/kg body weight, 48 h prior to mating with untreated females. The uterine contents of the females were evaluated for evidence of dominant lethal effects as manifested by an increase in the resorption rate. Among 1,2-dichloropropane-treated males, concentration-related decreases in water consumption were noted at all levels and decreased body weights were noted in males given 1 or 2.4 g/litre in the water. Mating performance was unaffected in these animals. Resorption rates among these groups revealed that the weekly values for the females mated to treated males ranged from 2.2 to 8.1%, well within the historical control range. Resorption rates among the concurrent controls were low, ranging from 3.5 to 5.4%. The significant increases from the concurrent control values, identified during the first week of breeding in the resorption rates in the groups given 0.24 or 2.4 g/litre, were considered to be within the normal variation. Cyclophosphamide resulted in a 10-fold increase in the resorption rate. 1,2-Dichloropropane was not mutagenic in a dominant lethal assay in male Sprague-Dawley rats exposed continuously to concentrations of up to 2.4 g/litre in the drinking-water (Hanley et al., 1989b).

8.4.2.3 Miscellaneous

Perocco et al. (1983) studied the tritiated thymidine uptake and cell viability in human lymphocyte cultures grown with, or without, rat liver metabolizing system. Both the [^{3}H]TdR uptake and the percentage of viable cells showed values very similar to control values. The 1,2-dichloropropane concentrations used ranged from 10^{-2} to 10^{-4} mmol/litre.

8.5 Carcinogenicity

8.5.1 Oral (mouse)

Groups of 7 to 9-week-old hybrid $B_6C_3F_1$ mice (50 males and 50 females) were administered 0, 125, or 250 mg 1,2-dichloropropane (99.4%)/kg body weight, in corn oil, by gavage, 5 days/week for 113 weeks. No influence on growth was observed. The survival of the female animals at the highest dose level was significantly decreased. The incidence of non-neoplastic lesions showed lesions of the spleen (haemosiderosis and haematopoiesis were increased) in female mice at the highest dose level.

The incidences of neoplastic lesions are summarized in Table 21.

On the basis of the results of this study, the NTP concluded that 1,2-dichloropropane induces an increased incidence of liver tumours in male and female $B_6C_3F_1$ mice (Haseman et al., 1984; NTP, 1986). However, the Task Group noted that the incidences of liver adenomas and carcinomas in the treated groups were within the historical ranges of this species (Haseman et al., 1985). The increased incidence of thyroid tumours is equivocal.

Table 21. The incidence of neoplastic lesions in a mouse study with 1,2-dichloropropane[a]

	Sex	Control	125 mg/kg	250 mg/kg
Adenoma (liver)	male	7/35 (20%)	9/33 (27%)	15/35 (43%)
Carcinoma (liver)	male	8/35 (23%)	10/33 (30%)	9/35 (26%)
Adenoma and carcinoma (liver)	male	15/35 (43%)	18/33 (55%)	24/35 (69%)[b]
Adenoma (liver)	female	1/35 (3%)	5/29 (17%)	5/26 (19%)[b]
Carcinoma (liver)	female	1/35 (3%)	2/29 (7%)	2/26 (8%)
Adenoma and carcinoma (liver)	female	2/35 (6%)	7/29 (24%)[b]	7/26 (27%)[b]
Follicular cell adenoma and carcinoma (thyroid)	female	1/34 (3%)	0/27 (0%)	5/24 (21%)[b]
Alveolar/bronchiolar adenoma or carcinoma (lung)	female	5/35 (14%)	0/29 (0%)	1/26 (4%)
Squamous cell papillomas (forestomach)	male female	0/50 (0%) 0/50 (0%)	1/48 (2%) 2/50 (4%)	3/49 (6%) 2/50 (4%)[c]

[a] From: NTP (1986).
[b] $P = \leq 0.05 - > 0.001$.
[c] One high-dose female mouse had a squamous cell carcinoma.

8.5.2 Oral (rat)

Groups of 50 male and 50 female F344/N rats (aged 7-9 weeks) were administered, by gavage, 0, 125 or 250 (female) and 0, 62, or 125 mg (male) 1,2-dichloropropane (99.4%)/kg body weight, in corn oil, 5 days/week for 103 weeks. The highest dose level showed growth depression in both sexes. Survival of female rats at the high dose level was significantly lower. The incidence of non-neoplastic lesions was not significantly different from that in the controls, except for an increased incidence of foci of clear cell change and of necrosis in the liver in high-dose female rats.

The incidences of neoplastic lesions are summarized in Table 22. Apart from these tumours, squamous cell papillomas of the forestomach were found in 1 control male and 1 female rat. In high-dose females, there was an increased incidence of mammary gland adenocarcinomas, but not of mammary gland adenomas. Apart from these tumours, squamous cell papillomas of the forestomach were found in two high-dose females (not significantly increased compared to controls). There were no effects on tumour incidences in male rats (Haseman et al., 1984; NTP, 1986).

Table 22. The incidence of neoplastic lesions in a rat study with 1,2-dichloropropane[a]

	Sex	Control	62 mg/kg male 125 mg/kg female	125 mg/kg male 250 mg/kg female
Fibroadenoma (mammary gland)	female	14/37 (38%)	20/43 (47%)	5/16 (31%)
Adenocarcinoma (mammary gland)	female	1/37 (3%)	2/43 (5%)	4/16 (25%)[b]
Endometrial stromal polyps (uterine tumours)	female	8/37 (22%)	14/42 (33%)	6/16 (38%)[b]
Liver tumours	male female	3/50 (6%) 0/50 (0%)	3/50 (6%) 0/50 (0%)	2/50 (4%) 0/50 (0%)
Islet cell adenoma and carcinoma (pancreas)	male	4/38 (11%)	1/42 (2%)	5/41 (12%)

[a] From: NTP (1986).
[b] $P = \leq 0.05$.

8.6 Factors modifying toxicity

Weanling Wistar rats, fed for several weeks on low protein choline-deficient diets, were more susceptible to the effects of inhalation of 4660 mg 1,2-dichloropropane/m^3 than rats on a control diet. This increased susceptibility could be corrected by dietary supplements of 1-methionine or 1-cysteine plus choline chloride (Heppel et al., 1946).

8.7 Special studies

8.7.1 Liver

Groups of 5 male Wistar rats (200 g) were administered, i.p., 0, 10, 25, 50, 100, 250, or 500 mg 1,2-dichloropropane (97%)/kg body weight, in corn oil, for 5 days (once daily) or for 4 weeks (five days/week), or a single dose of 0, 50, 100, or 250 mg/kg body weight, to investigate the biochemical and histological liver changes. Reduced glutathione (GSH), glutathione-S-transferase, cytochrome P450, and protein contents were measured. A dose-dependent decrease in liver-reduced glutathione was observed after a single injection and a dose-dependent increase after 4 weeks. The liver biochemical pattern after 4 weeks, characterized by a decrease of cytochrome P450 and by an increase in reduced glutathione and glutathione-S-transferase activity, suggests a hyperplastic evolution of the liver cells, probably a repair mechanism induced by the early depletion of glutathione. Histologically, the alterations confirm the regenerative nature (atypical mitosis and hyperplastic nodules) of the changes (Trevisan et al., 1989).

The hepatotoxicity of 1,2-dichloropropane (97%) in adult male Wistar rats (5 per group) was studied following daily i.p. injection at dose-levels of 0, 50, 100, 250, or 500 mg/kg body weight per day, in corn oil, for 4 weeks. Biochemical changes in the liver were demonstrated. Significant findings included reduction of aminopyrine demethylase activity at 100 mg/kg or more, increased levels of reduced glutathione and glutathione-S-transferase activity at 50 mg/kg or more, and decreased cytochrome P450 activity at 500 mg/kg. The activity of aniline hydroxylase was not affected. Duplicate groups of rats treated with 1,2-dichloropropane, but allowed a period of 4 weeks of recovery before being subjected to examination, showed that the induced biochemical changes in the liver were completely reversible (Trevisan et al., 1991).

1,2-Dichloropropane toxicity is actually preferentially mediated by GSH depletion. This is suggested by the fact that GSH loss is correlated with an increase in the biochemical indices of liver and renal injury, and with the extent of haemolysis.

Pretreatment of 1,2-dichloropropane-intoxicated rats with buthionine-sulfoximine (BSO) (depleting GSH) markedly increased the overall mortality. Furthermore, the administration of the GSH precursor *N*-acetyl-cysteine (NAC), preventing GSH depletion, reduced the damage in target tissues, as demonstrated by a smaller increase in some biochemical indices of cell injury and a smaller degree of haemolysis. A possible explanation for these findings is that, when the GSH level falls below a certain threshold value, irrespective of the causative agent, a series of common reactions is triggered, inducing peroxidation of membrane lipids, disturbances of Ca_2 homeostasis, and DNA damage, which quickly lead to irreversible liver injury. Furthermore, it is also possible that electrophilic metabolites of 1,2-dichloropropane, formed in the absence of GSH, could directly attack a variety of cell macromolecules the function of which is essentially to ensure the physiological survival of the hepatocytes (Mitchell et al., 1973; Bellomo & Orrenius, 1985; Casini et al., 1987; Orrenius et al., 1989).

Male Wistar rats were exposed (by gavage) to a single oral dose of 55 mg 1,2-dichloropropane/kg body weight in propylene glycol. The animals were killed 1-6 days after exposure. Glutathione (GSH), lipid peroxidation and protein of liver homogenate were measured. Reduction of hepatic GSH and total protein and enhanced hepatic lipid peroxidation still persisted 6 days after 1,2-dichloropropane administration (Di Nucci et al., 1988).

Groups of rats were treated orally, by gavage, with single doses of 1,2-dichloropropane ranging from 55 to 400 mg/kg body weight. 1,2-Dichloropropane was no longer detectable in the blood 24 h after dosing at any dose level (Di Nucci et al., 1988).

8.7.2 *Kidneys*

Renal failure caused by 1,2-dichloropropane has been reported by several authors who found an increase in serum creatinine and urea in intoxicated animals and humans and fatty degeneration or acute tubular damage in the kidney parenchyma (Heppel et al., 1946, Ponticelli et al., 1968; Pozzi et al., 1985; Imberti et al., 1987).

Imberti et al. (1990) suggested that, on the basis of the demonstration of 1,2-dichloropropane-induced depletion of kidney GSH, it may be postulated that the biochemical mechanisms involved in liver toxicity may also apply to the kidneys (Brezis et al., 1983). In addition, since most of the glutathione and cysteine conjugates of 1,2-dichloropropane are recovered in the urine, a direct toxicity of the conjugates to the kidneys seems to play an important role, as previously demonstrated for other conjugates (Stevens et al., 1988).

It has been demonstrated that GSH plays an essential role in the maintenance of the physiological structure of the erythrocyte, preventing the formation of inter-protein or intra-protein disulfides within the membrane skeleton. Depletion of erythrocyte glutathione causes an increased fragility of this cell and subsequent haemolysis. The involvement of such a mechanism in 1,2-dichloropropane-induced haemolysis in intoxicated animals is supported by the demonstration of a concomitant loss in erythrocyte GSH and a correlation between these 2 phenomena (Imberti et al., 1990).

Nephrotoxicity of 1,2-dichloropropane (97%) in adult male Wistar rats (5 per group) was studied following daily i.p. injection at dose levels of 0, 50, 100, 250, or 500 mg/kg body weight per day for 4 weeks. Biochemical and histopathological alterations of the kidneys were demonstrated. Kidney pathology involved a decrease in the activity of angiotensin-converting enzyme in the proximal tubule brush border and fraying of microvilli with epithelial coagulative necrosis. Duplicate groups of rats treated similarly with 1,2-dichloropropane, but allowed a period of 4 weeks of recovery before being subjected to examination, showed that the treatment-induced biochemical changes in the kidneys were completely reversible (Trevisan et al., 1988, 1991).

8.7.3 Central nervous system

In the study of Gorzinski & Johnson (1989), in which Fischer 344 rats were treated with 0, 300, or 500 mg 1,2-dichloropropane per kg body weight, by gavage, for 14 days, motor activity and a functional observational battery (unusual responses in behaviour, presence of convulsions, tremors, etc., and sensory function) were evaluated (section 8.2.1.2). No effects were seen on these parameters.

Specific tests in groups of 15 Fischer 344 rats/sex given, by gavage, 0 (corn oil), 20, 65, or 200 mg 1,2-dichloropropane (99.9%)/kg body weight, 5 days/week for 13 weeks, included monthly evaluation of a functional observation battery, hind limb grip strength, and motor activity; a comprehensive neuropathology study was carried out at the end of the study. Clinical observations included measurement of body weight gain and body temperature. Body weights were decreased for male rats given 200 mg/kg body weight. The body temperature was within normal limits, except in the females given 200 mg/kg, which showed a slightly lower temperature. No functional effects were noted. No gross or histopathological effects on either the central or peripheral nervous system were observed (Johnson & Gorzinski, 1988).

9. EFFECTS ON HUMANS

9.1 General population exposure

9.1.1 Acute toxicity - poisoning incidents

Ingestion of cleaning solvent (50 ml) containing 1,2-dichloropropane (other components not known) by a man produced coma followed by delirium, irreversible shock, cardiac failure, and death. Histopathologically, centri- and medio-lobular hepatic necrosis was found (Larcan et al., 1977).

Two cases of disseminated intravascular coagulation syndrome (DIC) have been described in association with acute intoxication by 1,2-dichloropropane. Effects on the central nervous system, liver, and kidney functions were also observed, but no details were given (Perbellini et al., 1985).

Pozzi et al. (1985), from Italy, reported clinical observations on 3 other hospitalized persons with 1,2-dichloropropane poisoning. Two out of the 3 persons ingested the substance, while the third person was exposed through inhalation. The clinical symptoms were similar, despite different routes of exposure. All 3 suffered from acute renal and hepatic damage. Kidney biopsy, carried out on 1 person, showed acute tubular necrosis. Haemolytic anaemia and disseminated intravascular coagulation were noted in all 3 patients, 1 of whom died on the seventh day. The other patients recovered after treatment.

Toxic hepatitis with portal hypertension has been described in a 49-year-old man, who ingested 1,2-dichloropropane in an attempted suicide (Thorel et al., 1986).

9.2 Occupational exposure

Baruffini et al. (1989) studied 10 cases of 1,2-dichloropropane dermatitis in the period 1985-88. Patients were painters or metalworkers in the engineering industry and they all had known contact with mixtures of solvents containing 10-40% 1,2-dichloropropane. On examination, the workers had itchy erythematous, oedematous, vesicular lesions on the fingers and dorsa of the hands. Two subjects also had scaling and fissuring of the palms. Cessation of exposure produced quick resolution of the dermatitis in all subjects. Patch tests were carried out. As controls, 120 subjects were similarly tested with 1,2-dichloropropane. All patients showed a positive response to concentrations of 2% 1,2-dichloropropane or more (allergic contact dermatitis). The results of the tests on the control subjects were negative.

Grzywa & Rudzki (1981) described cases of dermatitis in 2 women (47 and 55 years old), in a group of 60 persons, who had been exposed to Silform aerosols for 6 and 4 years, respectively. Silform aerosols contained 7.4, 11.0, or 12.7% 1,2-dichloropropane; methylsilicone oils, and Freon. The patch tests that were carried out were positive for 1,2-dichloropropane, but negative for methylsilicone oils.

10. PREVIOUS EVALUATIONS BY INTERNATIONAL BODIES

1,2-Dichloropropane was considered by working groups of the International Agency for Research on Cancer (IARC) in 1986 (IARC, 1986) and in 1987 (IARC, 1987). In the updating of 1987, it was evaluated as follows: "There is limited evidence for the carcinogenicity of 1,2-dichloropropane in experimental animals. There are no data in humans. The agent is not classifiable as to its carcinogenicity to humans (Group 3)".

WHO (in preparation) has proposed a provisional guideline value for drinking-water of 20 µg 1,2-dichloropropane/litre.

PART C

ENVIRONMENTAL HEALTH CRITERIA

FOR

MIXTURES OF DICHLOROPROPENES AND DICHLOROPROPANE

CONTENTS

ENVIRONMENTAL HEALTH CRITERIA FOR MIXTURES OF DICHLOROPROPENES AND DICHLOROPROPANE

1. SUMMARY AND EVALUATION, CONCLUSIONS, AND RECOMMENDATIONS 167

    1.1 Summary and evaluation 167
        1.1.1 Use, environmental fate, and environmental levels 167
        1.1.2 Kinetics and metabolism 167
        1.1.3 Effects on organisms in the environment 168
        1.1.4 Effects on experimental animals and *in vitro* test systems 168
        1.1.5 Effects on humans 169
    1.2 Conclusions 169
    1.3 Recommendations 170

2. IDENTITY, PHYSICAL AND CHEMICAL PROPERTIES, ANALYTICAL METHODS 171

    2.1 Identity 171
    2.2 Physical and chemical properties 171
    2.3 Analytical methods 172

3. SOURCES OF HUMAN AND ENVIRONMENTAL EXPOSURE 173

    3.1 Natural occurrence 173
    3.2 Man-made sources 173
    3.3 Uses 173

4. ENVIRONMENTAL TRANSPORT, DISTRIBUTION, AND TRANSFORMATION 174

    4.1 Air 174
    4.2 Water 174
    4.3 Soil 174
        4.3.1 Microbial transformation 174
        4.3.2 Loss under field conditions 174
        4.3.3 Soil function 176
    4.4 Bioconcentration 176

5.	ENVIRONMENTAL LEVELS AND HUMAN EXPOSURE		177
	5.1 Groundwater		177
	5.2 Occupational exposure		177
6.	KINETICS AND METABOLISM		178
7.	EFFECTS ON ORGANISMS IN THE ENVIRONMENT		179
	7.1 Microorganisms		179
	7.1.1 Terrestrial microorganisms		179
	7.1.1.1 Effects on nitrification		180
	7.1.1.2 Recovery studies with microorganisms		181
	7.2 Aquatic organisms		183
	7.2.1 Invertebrates		183
	7.2.2 Fish		183
	7.3 Terrestrial organisms		184
	7.3.1 Birds		184
	7.3.2 Soil fauna		184
	7.3.3 Plants		185
8.	EFFECTS ON EXPERIMENTAL ANIMALS AND *IN VITRO* TEST SYSTEMS		186
	8.1 Single exposures		186
	8.1.1 Oral		186
	8.1.2 Inhalation		186
	8.1.3 Dermal		186
	8.2 Short-term exposures		188
	8.2.1 Oral		188
	8.2.1.1 Rat		188
	8.2.1.2 Dog		188
	8.2.2 Inhalation		189
	8.3 Skin and eye irritation; sensitization		190
	8.3.1 Skin and eye irritation		190
	8.3.2 Sensitization		191
	8.4 Long-term exposures/carcinogenicity		191
	8.4.1 Oral		191
	8.4.1.1 Rat		191
	8.5 Reproduction, embryotoxicity, and teratogenicity		192
	8.5.1 Reproduction		192
	8.5.1.1 Oral		192
	8.5.1.2 Inhalation		193
	8.5.2 Embryotoxicity and teratogenicity		194
	8.5.2.1 Oral		194

8.6 Mutagenicity and related end-points 195
  8.6.1 *In vitro* studies (microorganisms) 195
  8.6.2 *In vivo* studies 195

9. EFFECTS ON HUMANS 197

  9.1 General population exposure 197
  9.2 Occupational exposure 197

1. SUMMARY AND EVALUATION, CONCLUSIONS AND RECOMMENDATIONS

1.1 Summary and evaluation

1.1.1 Use, environmental fate, and environmental levels

The technical mixture of dichloropropenes and dichloropropane (abbreviated in this text to "MIX D/D") is a clear amber liquid with a pungent odour; it has a vapour pressure of 35 mmHg at 20 °C, and is soluble in halogenated solvents, esters, and ketones.

"MIX D/D" typically contains not less than 50% 1,3-dichloropropene (ratio of *cis*- and *trans*-isomers approximately 1:1), the other main constituents being 1,2-dichloropropane and related compounds. It was widely used as a soil nematocide before planting.

The environmental transport, distribution, and fate of the major constituents of "MIX D/D" in air, water, and soil is described in the sections 4 of the parts of this EHC monograph that deal with 1,3-dichloropropene and 1,2-dichloropropane.

There is a significant potential for 1,2-dichloropropane derived from "MIX D/D" to leach from the soil and contaminate well water and groundwater. In an irrigation bore (68 m deep) in Western Europe, mean 1,2-dichloropropane concentrations at different depths ranged between 0.8 and 8.5 µg/litre, and the maximum concentration recorded was 165 µg/litre.

Significant uptake of the constituents of "MIX D/D" by crops is unlikely (see other parts of this EHC monograph). Bioaccumulation of the constituents of "MIX D/D" is also unlikely because of their low log P octanol/water partition coefficient and their relatively high water solubility.

1.1.2 Kinetics and metabolism

No metabolic studies have been carried out on "MIX D/D". The two major components, 1,3-dichloropropene and 1,2-dichloropropane, are rapidly eliminated, primarily in the urine and, to a lesser extent, via expired air. The components of "MIX D/D" are metabolized by oxidative and conjunction pathways. The major urinary metabolites are mercapturic acids.

1.1.3 Effects on organisms in the environment

"MIX D/D" is moderately toxic for fish; 96-h LC_{50} values range between 1 and 6 mg/litre. The 1,3-dichloropropene is largely responsible for the toxicity of "MIX D/D".

When used at recommended application rates, the main effects of "MIX D/D" are a transient (< 7 days) reduction in soil fungi and inhibition of the oxidation of ammonium ions to nitrate. "MIX D/D" is toxic for nitrifying bacteria. Soon after "MIX D/D" disappears from the soil, recolonization by bacteria takes place. In field trials, "MIX D/D" (applied at 600 litre/ha) killed soil invertebrates. Recolonization times ranged between 6 and 24 months.

"MIX D/D" is highly phytotoxic.

1.1.4 Effects on experimental animals and in vitro test systems

The acute toxicity of "MIX D/D" for laboratory animals is moderate to high. The oral LD_{50} values in rats and mice range from 132 to 300 mg/kg body weight. The dermal LD_{50} values for rats and rabbits are 779 and 2100 mg/kg body weight, respectively. The inhalation LC_{50} (4 h) for rats is approximately 4540 mg/m^3. Acute exposure results in clinical signs associated with central nervous system depression. "MIX D/D" is a severe eye and skin irritant and it is a moderate dermal sensitizer.

The results of the available short-term toxicity studies in rats and dogs are inadequate to assess properly the toxicity potential of "MIX D/D", because the relatively low doses tested do not demonstrate any biologically significant effects. Several short-term inhalation (whole-body) studies have been conducted in rats. "MIX D/D" at levels up to 145 mg/m^3 does not cause any toxic effects. At levels of 1362 mg/m^3 or higher, toxic effects associated with central nervous system depression are evident. An exposure to 443 mg/m^3 for 10 weeks leads to reduced body weight gain and increased absolute kidney weight.

An oral teratology study in rats was inadequate for assessment of the teratological potential of "MIX D/D".

In an inhalation rat study to investigate male and female fertility, no effects were found at dose levels up to 443 mg/m^3 for 10 weeks. Complete evaluation of reproductive effects of "MIX D/D" was not possible owing to inadequate protocol designs.

"MIX D/D" is mutagenic in *Salmonella typhimurium* strains TA100 and TA1535, as well as in *Escherichia coli* WP2 HCR, without metabolic activation. There was no such effect in *Salmonella* strains TA98, TA1537, and TA1538.

In a long-term study on rats fed diets containing up to 120 mg "MIX D/D" per kg (equivalent to 6 mg/kg body weight) for 2 years, no toxic or carcinogenic effects were seen.

1.1.5 Effects on humans

"MIX D/D" is no longer widely used, and, thus, exposure of the general population via air, water, and food is unlikely.

The exposure of workers filling drums and of field applicators was generally below 4.5 mg 1,3-dichloropropene/m^3 when recommended procedures were used; in other situations, levels up to 36.32 mg/m^3 have been measured.

One case of acute fatal poisoning has been reported following accidental ingestion of "MIX D/D".

Several cases of contact dermatitis and skin sensitization due to "MIX D/D" exposure have been reported.

1.2 Conclusions

- **General population.** As "MIX D/D" is no longer widely used, the exposure of the general population to 1,3-dichloropropene via air, water, and food is negligible, but, in certain areas, exposure to 1,2-dichloropropane may occur when groundwater is contaminated.

- **Occupational exposure.** Filling operations and field applications of "MIX D/D" can lead to exposure of operators to 1,3-dichloropropene that exceed maximum allowable concentrations, especially under warm climatic conditions.

- **Environment.** "MIX D/D" is unlikely to reach biologically significant levels in either the terrestrial or the aquatic environment when used at the recommended rate. Lasting adverse effects on organisms in the environment are unlikely to occur.

1.3 Recommendations

- "MIX D/D" should not be used as a soil fumigant because of potential leaching to groundwater.

- Monitoring of residues in surface water and groundwater should be carried out in areas where "MIX D/D" has been used.

2. IDENTITY, PHYSICAL AND CHEMICAL PROPERTIES, ANALYTICAL METHODS

2.1 Identity

The technical mixture of dichloropropenes and dichloropropane (abbreviated to "MIX D/D") contains not less than 50% of the *cis*- and *trans*-isomers (ratio approximately 1:1) of 1,3-dichloropropene and the other main constituent was 1,2-dichloropropane. Yang (1986) described a commercial "MIX D/D" containing 25% *cis*-dichloropropene, 27% of *trans*-dichloropropene, 29% 1,2-dichloropropane, and 19% other related chlorinated hydrocarbons. It may also contain 1% epichlorohydrin as a stabilizer.

CAS registry number: 8003-19-8.

For the physical and chemical properties of the main constituents, see the sections 2.2 of the parts of this monograph dealing with 1,3-dichloropropene and 1,2-dichloropropane.

Major trade names are D-D mixture, Nemafene, Nemax, Vidden-D.

Other formulations on the market are Ditrapex and Vortex (mixtures of 1,2-dichloropropane, 1,3-dichloropropene, and methylisothiocyanate), Ditrapex CP (the same mixture as Ditrapex, but also containing chloropicrin).

2.2 Physical and chemical properties

Technical "MIX D/D" is a clear amber liquid with a pungent odour. It has a vapour pressure of 4.6 kPa (20 °C) (35 mmHg at 20 °C), flash distils over the range of 59-115 °C, and has a relative density of 1.17-1.22 g/cm^3 at 20 °C; its flash point is 17.5 °C. Its solubility at room temperature is approximately 2 g/kg in water, but it is soluble at room temperature in hydrocarbon and halogenated solvents, esters, and ketones. The mixture is stable up to 500 °C (therefore stabilizers are not needed) but reacts with dilute organic bases, concentrated acids, halogens, and some metal salts. It is corrosive to some metals (e.g., aluminium, magnesium, and their alloys, and may remove lacquer from lacquer-lined containers. It is not corrosive to mild steel.

2.3 Analytical methods

The same methods can be used as for 1,3-dichloropropene.

See section 2.4 of the part of this monograph that deals with 1,3-dichloropropene.

3. SOURCES OF HUMAN AND ENVIRONMENTAL EXPOSURE

3.1 Natural occurrence

"MIX D/D" does not occur naturally.

3.2 Man-made sources

"MIX D/D" is manufactured by high temperature chlorination of propene.

For sources of pollution, see section 3.2.3 of the part of this monograph that deals with 1,3-dichloropropene and section 3.2 of 1,2-dichloropropane.

3.3 Uses

"MIX D/D" is a preplant nematocide, effective against soil nematodes including root knot, meadow, sting and dagger, spiral, and sugar beet nematodes. It is usually applied by injection into the soil or through tractor-drawn hollow tines, to a depth of 15-20 cm at a rate of 150-400 litre/ha (occasionally to a maximum of 1000 litre/ha), depending on soil type and the following crop. The soil surface is sealed by rolling. "MIX D/D" volatilizes and diffuses as a vapour and, thus, its effectiveness depends on how readily this can occur. Because the components of "MIX D/D" are highly phytotoxic, it is essential that, after an application of 220 litre/ha or more, a period of not less than 14 days should elapse before planting or sowing (Shell, 1985).

4. ENVIRONMENTAL TRANSPORT, DISTRIBUTION, AND TRANSFORMATION

4.1 Air

(See section 4 of 1,3-dichloropropene and 1,2-dichloropropane).

4.2 Water

(See section 4 of 1,3-dichloropropene and 1,2-dichloropropane).

4.3 Soil

(See section 4 of 1,3-dichloropropene and 1,2-dichloropropane).

4.3.1 Microbial transformation

It has been demonstrated under *in vitro* and *in vivo* conditions that indigenous soil microflora can utilize C3 chlorinated hydrocarbons. Four species, *Bacillus subtilis, Arthrobacter globiformis, Pseudomonas fluorescens*, and *Rhizobium leguminosarum*, were successfully grown on media including "MIX D/D" (Altman & Lawlor, 1966; Altman, 1969).

Toxicity tests were carried out with *Rhizobium phaseoli* and *Azotobacter beinjerinckii*, both nitrogen-fixing bacteria, in cultures using unsterilized Hanford sandy loam. "MIX D/D" at concentrations ranging from 10 to 100 mg/kg and 100 to 1000 mg/kg caused growth inhibition in *Azotobacter beinjerinckii* and *Rhizobium phaseoli*, respectively (Rader & Love, 1977a).

4.3.2 Loss under field conditions

A trial has been carried out in the United Kingdom in which "MIX D/D" was applied at 410 litre/ha (see section 4.1.3.5 of 1,3-dichloropropene). Samples of soil were taken at 3 depths: 0-20 cm, 20-40 cm, and 40-60 cm, at 6 intervals up to $9\frac{1}{2}$ months after application. The results are summarized in Table 23. Residues of 1,3-dichloropropenes, 1,2-dichloropropane, and 3-chloroallyl alcohols were present in all 3 soil layers, especially before ploughing. They showed little change in the period before ploughing, but, thereafter, the concentrations decreased gradually (Wallace, 1979).

Table 23. Residues from the plot treated with "Mix D/D" at 410 litre/ha

Interval since application (days)	Soil depth (cm)	Concentration in soil (mg/kg)				
		1,3-dichloro-propenes		1,2-dichloro-propane	3-chloroallyl alcohols	
		cis-isomer	trans-isomer		cis-isomer	trans-isomer
3	0-20	6.82	6.05	8.7	2.02	1.98
	20-40	6.83	7.08	9.8	1.36	1.35
	40-60	0.85	0.90	1.4	0.24	0.24
11	0-20	3.50	3.50	5.4	0.63	0.53
	20-40	4.84	5.05	6.5	1.86	2.11
	40-60	0.35	0.35	0.9	0.18	0.17
24	0-20	5.73	5.55	9.4	1.0	1.0
	20-40	6.07	6.21	12.5	2.0	2.0
	40-60	0.70	0.63	2.1	0.29	0.29
33		NORMAL CULTIVATION (ploughing of the soil)				
40	0-20	0.73	0.86	0.77	0.58	0.44
	20-40	1.54	1.79	1.90	0.41	0.37
	40-60	0.30	0.30	1.00	0.14	0.15
73	0-20	0.26	0.25	0.2	0.16	0.11
	20-40	0.64	0.62	1.5	0.36	0.28
	40-60	0.51	0.44	2.9	0.22	0.19
At harvest 9½ months	0-20	0.06	0.05	0.1	0.16	0.08
	20-40	0.03[a]	0.02[a]	0.2	0.07	0.03
	40-60	< 0.01	< 0.01	0.2	< 0.02	< 0.02
Pre-treatment	0-20	< 0.01	< 0.01	< 0.1	< 0.02	< 0.02
	20-40	< 0.01	< 0.01	< 0.1	< 0.02	< 0.02
	40-60	< 0.01	< 0.01	< 0.1	< 0.02	< 0.02

[a] Results confirmed by GC/MS.
From: Wallace (1979).
Note: All residues are on a dry weight basis.

4.3.3 Soil function

"MIX D/D" soil fumigant, 337 and 3370 kg active ingredient per ha, was used to evaluate the effect on nodulation of pinto bean plants in soil and on the growth of root nodule bacteria in culture. Unsterilized Hanford sandy loam was used. After 4 weeks' growing time, low and high doses of "MIX D/D" resulted in a reduction in root nodules of approximately 70 and 80%, respectively; the percentages of germination were about 90 and 50%, respectively (Rader & Love, 1977a).

Unsterilized Oakdale loamy sand soil (81.6% sand, 11.2% silt and 1.06% organic carbon), treated with "MIX D/D" soil fumigant at 337 and 1348 kg active ingredient/ha, in 1978, showed no decrease in soil phosphatase activity after 0, 4, and 8 weeks at an incubation temperature of 27 °C (Rader, 1979c).

The effects were studied of "MIX D/D" soil fumigant (337 and 3370 kg/ha) on proteolytic enzyme activity in the treated soil. The soil proteases were assayed by the release of tyrosine from sodium caseinate in the treated soil, after incubation periods of 0, 4, 8, and 12 weeks, at 27 °C. No inhibitory effects were found (Rader, 1979b).

"MIX D/D", at a high dose of 100-1000 mg/kg, caused a temporary loss of cellulytic activity in *Trichoderma viride* (Rader & Love, 1977b).

Laboratory studies were conducted to determine the effects of "MIX D/D" on the activities of invertase in a sandy soil. The rates of application were 150 and 300 mg/kg. No inhibition was found. The same dose levels were used to study the influence of "MIX D/D" on amylase activity in this soil. After 3 days, stimulation of glucose formation from the added starch was observed, especially at the lowest dose level. Microbial respiration was also studied. The treatments did not significantly decrease oxygen consumption (Tu, 1988).

4.4 Bioconcentration

No data on bioconcentration are available.

5. ENVIRONMENTAL LEVELS AND HUMAN EXPOSURE

Analyses have been made to determine whether residues of the active 1,3-dichloropropene isomers could be found in the edible parts of a number of crops, including potatoes, carrots, onions, cucurbits, rice, and sugar beet. At recommended rates and pre-planting intervals, residues of these propenes (*cis-* and *trans-*isomers) have not been detected (limit of determination 0.02 mg/kg) (see section 2.4 of 1,3-dichloropropene).

5.1 Groundwater

1,2-Dichloropropane levels of 0.8-8.5 µg/litre, with a maximum of 165 µg/litre, were reported in groundwater in the Netherlands from bores for irrigation at depths up to 68 m. These levels resulted from previous applications of "MIX D/D" (Leistra & Boesten, 1989) (see section 5.1.2 of 1,2-dichloropropane).

5.2 Occupational exposure

Field studies were carried out in several locations in the Netherlands and in France to monitor personal exposure and environmental concentrations during application of "MIX D/D". In most of the 11 locations in the Netherlands, the time-weighted average of the exposure of the operators, as measured with personal sampler pumps during application, was of the order of 4.54 mg total *cis-* and *trans-*1,3-dichloropropene per m^3. When filling operations are carried out in the recommended way, personal exposures can be limited to a maximum of 4.54 mg/m^3. Levels of the unsaturated components of "MIX D/D" in the air 1 m above the soil surface shortly after application were below 0.454 mg/m^3.

In most of the 9 locations in France, the time-weighted average exposure levels of the operators, as measured with personal sampler pumps, was of the order of 4.54-9.08 mg total *cis-* and *trans-*1,3-dichloropropene per m^3. Peak exposures of up to 36.32 mg/m^3 were measured when the recommended safety precautions were insufficiently observed. Levels of the unsaturated components of "MIX D/D" in the air 1 m above the soil surface during application ranged from 1 to 6.4 mg/m^3 (van Sittert et al., 1977; van Sittert, 1978).

6. KINETICS AND METABOLISM

See section 6 in the parts of this monograph that deal with both 1,3-dichloropropene and 1,2-dichloropropane.

No information is available on the kinetics and metabolism of other compounds, impurities, and stabilizers that may be present in "MIX D/D".

7. EFFECTS ON ORGANISMS IN THE ENVIRONMENT

7.1 Microorganisms

(See also relevant sections of 1,3-dichloropropene and 1,2-dichloropropane.)

7.1.1 Terrestrial microorganisms

The effects of "MIX D/D" on microorganisms and on soil function have been widely studied in Europe (Pochon et al., 1951; Bakker, 1968; Sommer, 1970; Kämpfe, 1973; Lebbink & Kolenbrander, 1974), in Canada (Wensley, 1953; Elliot et al., 1972, 1974, 1977; Tu, 1972, 1973, 1978, 1979, 1981a,b), in the USA (Thornton, 1951; Moje et al., 1957), and elsewhere (Dommergues, 1959; Mehta et al., 1963; Dubey et al., 1975; Ross & McNeilly, 1975). Main interest has been in the microorganisms involved in the nitrogen balance of the soil, as this bears strongly upon the yields of crops grown in treated soil.

During the search for effective soil fumigants, the toxicity of "MIX D/D" for soil microorganisms has been investigated on 2 soil types, a sandy loam and a soil with high organic matter. At a dosage of 1200 mg/kg soil, the following reductions in soil microorganisms were found after 96 h: bacteria 90%, actinomycetes 99%, and fungi 98%. The toxicity of the major components of "MIX D/D" for these same major groups of microorganisms has been studied in soil samples from old citrus plantations under laboratory conditions, and it was found that the toxicity of 1,2-dichloropropane for fungi and bacteria and actinomycetes was low to moderate (Moje et al., 1957).

The studies of Wensley (1953) and of Moje et al. (1957) are reasonably consistent and indicate that bacteria are more tolerant to "MIX D/D" than fungi, and, again, that the toxicity of "MIX D/D" is related mainly to its 1,3-dichloropropene content, in particular the *cis*-isomer.

Rader et al. (1978) studied the correlation between the numbers of soil microorganisms and the O_2/CO_2 exchange in treated soil. Unsterilized Hanford sandy loam (57.6% sand, 26.6% silt, 15.8% clay, and 0.7% organic carbon) was used and the soil had a moisture content of 6%. "MIX D/D" soil fumigant (dosages 336 and 2240 kg active ingredient/ha) caused a decrease in the populations of actinomycetes, bacteria, and fungi, and also reduced the oxygen utilization by soil microorganisms.

7.1.1.1 Effects on nitrification

Kämpfe (1973) studied the inhibition by "MIX D/D" of nitrification in a black earth soil. Nitrogen (180 mg/kg, NH_3 and NH_3-water) and "MIX D/D" (80 mg/kg) were applied at different temperatures. The time of incubation was 30-120 days. At temperatures between 5 °C and 10 °C, nitrification of NH_3 was severely inhibited for 90 days. After 120 days of incubation at 10 °C, 70% of the nitrogen applied was retrieved as ammonium-ion.

The inhibition of ammonium nitrogen oxidation has led to the build-up of ammonium nitrogen in treated soil under both laboratory (Sommer, 1970) and field conditions (Thornton, 1951; Mehta et al., 1963; Elliot et al., 1974; Ross & McNeilly, 1975).

"MIX D/D" was extremely toxic to nitrifying bacteria in silty clay loam or loam soils. Doses of 200, 2000, and 20 000 mg "MIX D/D"/kg soil were tested. Inhibition of NH_4^+-oxidizing bacteria was found, but not of *Nitrobacter* spp. Nitrogen mineralization was progressively depressed with increasing levels of "MIX D/D". At 200 mg "MIX D/D"/kg soil, nitrate formation from ammonium nitrogen was very markedly reduced, while mineralization of nitrogen was only slightly reduced at 20 000 mg/kg soil (Dubey et al., 1975). These results are in agreement with the results of Bromley & Cook (1981).

Bromley & Cook (1981) also studied the influence of "MIX D/D" on the nitrification processes in soil. Transient inhibition of nitrification (< 20 days) occurred in sandy clay treated with 200 or 1000 mg "MIX D/D"/kg. Considerable (80% reduction compared with controls) and total inhibition occurred in soil treated with 2000 and 10 000 mg "MIX D/D"/kg, respectively. There was no difference between the inhibitory effects of "MIX D/D" and those of a purified dichloropropene isomer mixture, indicating that the dichloropropenes were the active inhibitors in "MIX D/D". During inhibition of nitrification by "MIX D/D", ammonium accumulated but no significant nitrite accumulation was observed. This indicates that ammonification was unaffected and that inhibition of nitrification resulted from the specific inhibition of *Nitrosomonas* spp. Overall, it was concluded that "MIX D/D" was not very active as a nitrification inhibitor, compared with commercially available inhibitors.

Unsterilized Handford sandy loam was fumigated with "MIX D/D" soil fumigant. The soil was moistened to 75% moisture content, and was composed as follows: 0.7% organic carbon, 57.5% sand, 26.6% silt, and 15.8% clay. The activity of the nitrifying bacteria (oxidation of nitrite-nitrogen to nitrate-nitrogen) was monitored. After the treated soil had been incubated for 1-4 months at 27 °C, nitrite could not be detected. "MIX D/D" soil fumigant did reduce the oxidation of the ammonia to nitrite by *Nitrosomonas* spp., especially at a concentration four times normal field use. There was no effect on *Nitrobacter* spp. (Rader, 1979a).

"MIX D/D" application kills a considerable part of the biomass. Lysis of the killed biomass provides the surviving microflora with a new and, to some extent, readily available substrate. The mineralization of this substrate, together with a small priming effect, gives an extra contribution to the inorganic nitrogen content of the soil (so-called "flush"). This contribution depends on the amount of biomass, which is related to the type of soil. The gain in nitrogen is approximately 5-10 kg N/ha. The nitrogen gain in spring, after autumn fumigation, can be attributed to a reduction in loss of nitrogen by diminished leaching and diminished denitrification of nitrate, and depends on the rate of mineralization, time of recovery of nitrification, weather conditions during the winter, and soil type (Lebbink & Kolenbrander, 1974).

In field trials, the influence of "MIX D/D" on nitrification was studied in loamy sand and black earth soils. Nitrogen application was 100 kg/ha; and the application of "MIX D/D" was between 37.1 and 46.6 kg/ha. When "MIX D/D" had been applied to the loamy sand, 61.5% of the September-applied nitrogen was retrieved in the top 20 cm in March of the following year. This percentage went up to 72 and 100%, respectively, when fertilizer was applied in October or November. On loamy sand, the yield obtained from the following crop was significantly increased. On black earth, "MIX D/D" application resulted in only a slight increase in crop yield (Kämpfe, 1973).

7.1.1.2 Recovery studies with microorganisms

"MIX D/D" was added to soil at 2 rates, approximately 10 and 100 times the normal recommended treatment rates. A number of microbial assessments were made (see below).

Parameter	% reduction over control at:	
	3000 litre/ha	30 000 litre/ha
Evolution of carbon dioxide	10	100
Density of total bacteria	nd[a]	98
Density of proteolytic bacteria	44	99
Density of cellulolytic bacteria	30	100
Mineralization of nitrogen	9	44
Mineralization of asparagin	0	27

[a] Not determined.
From: Dommergues (1959).

Soon after the "MIX D/D" disappears from the soil, recolonization by bacteria takes place and the number of the different types of bacteria may be higher than before the "MIX D/D" treatment; this may lead to the production of higher levels of nitrogen/ha, perhaps because of a belated recovery of bacteriophages (Bakker, 1968).

With "MIX D/D" (120 and 600 mg/kg), Tu (1972) found a decrease in bacterial and fungal populations in a loamy sand, but recovery to the same levels as the controls was rapid. In a series of studies by Tu (1978, 1979, 1981a,b), "MIX D/D" at 150 and 300 mg/kg soil, and 1,3-dichloropropene at 30 and 60 mg/kg, were evaluated in parallel under laboratory conditions. In general, neither had much effect on either the numbers of soil microorganisms or their activity. Acetylene reduction, the population of non-symbiotic nitrogen-fixing organisms, and the viability of indigenous microorganisms were not affected. There was some stimulation of microbial numbers in some experiments. Soil enzyme activity was either not affected or only very slightly affected.

Overall, the main effect of "MIX D/D" on soil microbial function, at normal usage levels, is to reduce the rate of turnover of ammonium. After autumn treatment, this is an advantage, as ammonium leaches from the soil less readily than nitrate and so is available in the spring for crop growth (Elliot et al., 1974). This effect, together with increased chlorine content, contributes to the yield increases beyond those expected from pest control alone, that are often noted following "MIX D/D" treatment (Goffart & Heiling, 1958; Ennik et al., 1964; Bakker, 1968).

7.2 Aquatic organisms

7.2.1 Invertebrates

Varanka (1979) studied the toxicity of "MIX D/D" (50% 1,3-dichloropropene + 1,2-dichloropropane) for the larvae (*glochidia*) of freshwater mussels (*Anodonta cygnea* L.). The decrease of tryptamine-induced adductor muscle activity was used as an indicator of the effect of the pesticide. The presence of toxicants reduces the ability of the larval adductor muscle to contract when stimulated by tryptamine. In each experiment, 200-300 larvae originating from 4-5 adult mussels were used. The concentration of "MIX D/D" causing 50% reduction in adductor muscle activity, over a 30-min exposure, was 18 mg/litre (20 ppm v/v).

7.2.2 Fish

"MIX D/D" is moderately toxic for fish (Table 24). The toxicity is largely due to the 1,3-dichloropropene component, 1,2-dichloropropane being about two orders of magnitude less toxic than "MIX D/D" (see section 7.1.3 of 1,2-dichloropropane).

Harlequin fish (*Rasbora heteromorpha*) were exposed in water containing 10 mg "MIX D/D"/litre. After 2 h, no deaths were found. The fish were then transferred to clean water and 3 days later there were still no deaths. In another study, 5 fish were exposed continuously in water containing 5 mg "MIX D/D"/litre. Three fish had died by 45 h, but no further deaths had occurred by 96 h (Reiff, 1975).

Application of "MIX D/D" (1000 litre/ha) to a vineyard in France caused contamination of a natural spring, which in turn led to contamination of fish-breeding basins and a pond. "MIX D/D" was detected in the spring water 20 days after the death of trout and carp. The concentrations in the spring and pond water ranged from 0.4 to 2.4 mg/litre. Within 3 months, the concentration decreased to less than 0.1 mg/litre (Elgar et al., 1965).

Table 24. Acute toxicity of "Mix D/D" to fish

Species	Size	Temperature (°C)	96-h LC_{50} (mg/litre)	References
Rainbow trout (*Oncorhynchus mykiss*)	1.1 g	12	5.5[a] (3.6-8.4)	Mayer & Ellersieck (1986)
	1.1 g	12	1.97[b] (1.2-3.2)	
Cutthroat trout (*Salmo clarki*)	1.0 g	12	1-10	Mayer & Ellersieck (1986)
Walleye (*Stizostedion vitreum*)	1.3 g	18	0.98[b]	Mayer & Ellersieck (1986)
Largemouth bass (*Micropterus salmoides*)	0.9 g	18	3.4[b]	Mayer & Ellersieck (1986)
Bluegill sunfish (*Lepomis macrochirus*)	1.4 g	18	3.9[b]	Mayer & Ellersieck (1986)
Channel catfish (*Ictalurus punctatus*)	1.1 g	18	4.4[b]	Mayer & Ellersieck (1986)
Harlequin fish (*Rasbora heteromorpha*)	2-3 cm	20-22[c]	4-5	Reiff (1975)
Carp (*Cyprimus carpio*)	-	-	6[d]	Reiff (1975)

[a] Water hardness, 44 mg $CaCO_3$/litre.
[b] Water hardness, 272 mg $CaCO_3$/litre.
[c] Hard, chlorine-free water (260 mg $CaCO_3$/litre).
[d] At 24 h.

7.3 Terrestrial organisms

7.3.1 Birds

No data were available.

7.3.2 Soil fauna

In one study in the United Kingdom, 99% of soil arthropods were killed following "MIX D/D" application. It took more than 2 years for the population to recover completely, although the chemical itself disappeared in about 4 weeks. *Collembola* populations started to build up again after 6 months and exceeded 50% of the initial population after 10 months. Populations were not monitored beyond 10 months (Edwards & Lofty, 1969).

Studies on a light sandy soil in Belgium showed somewhat faster recolonization rates. In an unreplicated experiment, 10-11 months after the last of 5 successive yearly treatments of 600 litre "MIX D/D"/ha, it was found that populations of phytophagous nematodes, but not of saprophagous nematodes, were depressed. Earthworms, enchytraeid worms, mites, and *Collembola* were present, mainly in the top 5 cm of the soil. Populations of these groups were not significantly depressed relative to the untreated plot. Populations of earthworms and mites were significantly increased (van den Brande & Heungens, 1969).

In a replicated study, the influence of four, successive, yearly applications of "MIX D/D" (600 litre/ha) on the soil fauna was studied in a sandy soil in which begonias were grown. Again, recolonization was found between 6 and 12 months after treatment. Of the groups studied 12 months after the last treatment, there was little or no effect on the populations of Enchytraeidae, *Gamasina*, Onychiuridae, Lumbricidae, and Acaridae. In the remaining 5 groups (of mites and *Collembola*), the populations were also similar to those in untreated plots (Heungens & van Daele, 1974).

7.3.3 Plants

The components of "MIX D/D" are highly phytotoxic.

8. EFFECTS ON EXPERIMENTAL ANIMALS AND IN VITRO TEST SYSTEMS

8.1 Single exposures

8.1.1 Oral

The acute oral toxicity of "MIX D/D" (containing 51.5% of 1,3-dichloropropene) was moderate to high when it was administered to mice, rats, and dogs (Table 25). Signs of intoxication in rats and mice were hyperexcitability, followed by incoordination, depression, dyspnoea, and chromodacryorrhoea. Most of the surviving animals had recovered within 24 h of dosing (Hine et al., 1953; Coombs & Carter, 1976a).

8.1.2 Inhalation

Long-Evans rats were exposed for 4 h in atmospheres containing 2043-81 720 mg "MIX D/D"/m^3. The animals were observed for 10 days. The LC_{50} was approximately 4540 mg/m^3. The rats that died showed severe oedema of the lung, with haemorrhages. Congestion, cloudy swelling, and fatty degeneration of the liver were also observed (Hine et al., 1952, 1953).

8.1.3 Dermal

The acute toxicity of "MIX D/D" is low when it is applied in a single percutaneous dose to rats. Signs of intoxication included lethargy and chromodacryorrhoea that disappeared in survivors within 4 days after dosing (Hine et al., 1953; Coombs & Carter, 1976a).

Nineteen adult rabbits were treated with 1.2-4.8 g "MIX D/D"/kg body weight, on the skin, for 24 h. Inhalation of the vapour was not possible. A mucous nasal discharge was noted in one rabbit treated with 3 g "MIX D/D"/kg body weight. The skin showed extremely severe eschar with intense oedema, resulting in black necrotic tissue. Seven of the 10 animals receiving the three higher dose levels died in 8-48 h. The LD_{50} was 2.1 g/kg body weight (see Table 25) (Hine et al., 1952, 1953).

Table 25. Acute toxicity of "Mix D/D"

Species	Route	Vehicle	Sex	LD_{50} (mg/kg body weight)[a]	References
Mouse (Swiss)	oral	propylene glycol	male	300	Hine et al. (1952, 1953)
Mouse (CD-1)	oral	undiluted		314 (276-365)	Coombs & Carter (1976a)
Mouse (CF-1)	oral	3% D-D in DMSO		234 (208-262)	Carter (1975)
Rat (Long-Evans)	oral	suspension in propylene glycol		140	Hine et al. (1952, 1953)
Rat (CD)	oral	undiluted	male female	227 (180-540) 132 (108-156)	Coombs & Carter (1976a)
Dog	oral	undiluted		> 230[b]	Carter (1975)
Rat (CD)	dermal	undiluted		779 (630-1103)	Coombs & Carter (1976a)
Rabbit	dermal	undiluted	male	2100 (1540-2660)	Hine et al. (1952, 1953)

[a] With 95% confidence limits.
[b] Screening value from test with only 2 dogs/dose. Apart from vomiting in dogs, no signs of intoxication were observed.

8.2 Short-term exposures

8.2.1 Oral

8.2.1.1 Rat

Carworth Farm E-rats (12 of each sex per group) were dosed orally, by gavage, with emulsions of "MIX D/D" in corn oil at 0, 0.0125, 0.025, 0.125, or 3.125 mg "MIX D/D"/kg body weight per day, for 3 months. The "MIX D/D" contained 55% 1,3-dichloropropenes, 26% 1,2-dichloropropane, and 0.7% epichlorohydrin. There were no effects on general health, behaviour, growth rate, food intake, or blood chemistry throughout the experiment. No changes in organ weights or pathological lesions attributable to "MIX D/D" were detected at any dose level.

When rats were dosed with 3.125 mg/kg body weight, there were slight reductions in the haemoglobin concentration and erythrocyte count in the males, and at 0.125 mg/kg body weight there were reductions in the erythrocyte and total leukocyte counts in the females, but since these reductions were not dose-related, they were of doubtful toxicological significance. With a dose of 0.025 mg/kg body weight there were no effects attributable to the "MIX D/D" (Walker, 1968a). (Remark: The Task Group noted that the dose levels used were too low for a proper assessment of the toxicity).

8.2.1.2 Dog

Beagle dogs (3 of each sex per dose group, with 5 of each sex as controls) were orally dosed by capsule with 0, 0.0125, 0.025, or 3.125 mg "MIX D/D"/kg body weight per day, for 3 months. The composition of the "MIX D/D" was 55% 1,3-dichloropropenes, 26% 1,2-dichloropropane, and 0.7% epichlorohydrin. There were no effects on general health, behaviour, growth rate, haematology, or clinical chemistry at any dose level. No pathological lesions attributable to "MIX D/D" were detected, even at the highest dose level (Walker, 1968b). (Remark: The Task Group noted that the dose levels used were too low for a proper assessment of the toxicity).

Groups of 4 pure-bred Beagle dogs and 4 bitches were dosed with 0, 0.25, 0.75, 2.50, or 7.50 mg/kg body weight "MIX D/D" (containing 28.2% *cis*-, 29.0% *trans*-1,3-dichloropropene, and 34.0% 1,2-dichloropropane, without epichlorohydrin), suspended in olive oil in gelatin capsules, 7 days/week, for 2 years. Haematological and blood chemistry studies and urinalyses were conducted on each animal just prior to the inception of the study and after 3, 6, 9, 12, 18, and 24 months of testing. Ten organs were weighed and histopathological examination was carried out of 28 organs and tissues.

The overall body weights of the bitches were lower in the 7.5 mg/kg group compared to untreated bitches. The mean corpuscular volume and mean corpuscular haemoglobin level were lower in the bitches of the 7.5 mg/kg group, while their erythrocyte count was raised above that of untreated bitches. No other effects were found. At the dose level of 2.5 mg/kg, no differences were found in the body weight, food intake, behaviour, mortality, haematology, clinical chemistry, urinalysis, organ weight, or gross or histopathological appearance between treated and control animals (Industr. Biotest Lab., 1977b). An audit of the study data concluded that no deviations from the protocol were observed which influenced the overall interpretation. Repeated oral dosing of dogs with 7.5 mg "MIX D/D"/kg body weight per day, for 2 years, did not result in any significant biological effects (Schweizer & Parker, 1980; Parker, 1980).

8.2.2 Inhalation

Male or female Long-Evans rats (6 per group) were exposed, whole body, in concentrations of 0, 340.5, 1362, or 2724 mg "MIX D/D"/m^3, 1 h/day, 5 days a week, for 2 weeks, or until the animals died. Rats exposed to the two highest dose levels showed evidence of weight loss, central nervous system depression, and moderate irritation. At 2724 mg/m^3, 3 animals died. There were no deaths in the other groups and no gross or microscopic lesions were observed. No effects were seen in the 340.5 mg/m^3 group (Hine et al., 1952). A further group of six rats was exposed to 1362 mg "MIX D/D"/m^3, 1 h/day, for 3 days. They were killed to find out whether there were any lesions immediately after exposure. No gross or microscopic lesions were found (Hine et al., 1952).

Groups of 28 male and 28 female Fischer 344 albino rats and CD-1 albino mice were exposed to atmospheres containing 0, 22.7, 68.1, or 227 mg "MIX D/D"/m^3, for 6 h/day, 5 days/week for 6 or 12 weeks. The actual mean concentrations were 0, 21.16, 65.38, and 243.8 mg/m^3. No unusual signs of toxicity were observed in rats or mice during the study. Body weights and mortality were similar in all groups at both 6 and 12 weeks. There were no treatment-related changes in haematology, clinical chemistry, or urinalysis apart from the detection of small to moderate amounts of occult blood in the urine of female mice exposed to 22.7, 68.1, or 227 mg "MIX D/D"/m^3 for 6 weeks. No treatment-related changes were observed in absolute organ weights of rats or mice exposed to "MIX D/D" atmospheres up to, and including, 227 mg/m^3, for 6 or 12 weeks. Small changes attributable to "MIX D/D" exposure were observed in male rats exposed to 227 mg/m^3 (increased liver/body weight ratio) at 6 and 12 weeks and in female rats exposed to 227 mg/m^3 (increased kidney/body weight ratio) at 12 weeks. No treatment-related histopathological changes were observed in either rats or mice, other than slight to moderate diffuse hepatocytic enlargement in male mice (12/21) after 12 weeks exposure to 227 mg "MIX D/D"/m^3. No significant changes related to toxicity were found in the body weight, behaviour, haematology, clinical chemistry, or gross or histological appearance of rats or mice exposed to atmospheres containing up to, and including, 227 mg "MIX D/D"/m^3, for 6 or 12 weeks. No adverse effects were seen at the top dose level (Hazleton Laboratories America Inc., 1979; Parker et al., 1982).

Groups of 30 male and 24 female Wistar SPF albino rats were exposed to actual concentrations of 0, 64, 145, or 443 mg "MIX D/D"/m^3, 6 h/day 5 days per week, for 10 weeks. The "MIX D/D" contained 28.1% *cis*-1,3-dichloropropene, 25.6% *trans*-1,3-dichloropropene, and 25.6% 1,2-dichloropropane, without epichlorohydrin. A subgroup was used for the reproduction study (see also section 8.5.1.2). There were no compound-related changes in the urinalysis, haematology, clinical chemistry, or in the gross or histological appearance of the reproductive tract in male and female rats. Males and females exposed to 443 mg "MIX D/D"/m^3 showed a reduced weight gain compared to controls, indicative of a mild toxic response at this top dose. Absolute kidney weights in females were higher in the 443 mg/m^3 group compared to controls, but apart from a slight increase in amorphous protein casts in the proximal convoluted tubular lumina, no histopathological effects were observed. This increase in kidney weight was probably related to the efficient renal excretion of "MIX D/D". A no-observed-effect level (NOEL) of 145 mg/m^3 was considered (Clark, 1980).

8.3 Skin and eye irritation; sensitization

8.3.1 Skin and eye irritation

Undiluted "MIX D/D" was applied to the skin of 12 rabbits in single doses of 0.5 ml. The liquid was allowed to be in contact with the skin for 24 h. The mean score was 7 on the scale (up to 8) of the method of Draize et al. (1944): rating it as a severe irritant. Signs were severe eschar, intense oedema, and black necrotic tissue (Hine et al., 1952, 1953; Coombs & Carter, 1976a).

Six young New Zealand albino rabbits were used in a primary skin-irritation test. 0.5 ml of undiluted "MIX D/D" soil fumigant was applied on the skin for 4 h. The mean scores for erythema and oedema after 4, 24, and 72 h were averaged. The primary irritation score was 8, rating it as corrosive. The signs were erythema, oedema, escharosis, and necrosis (Industr. Biotest Lab., 1972).

Undiluted "MIX D/D" was instilled into the eyes of 10 rabbits in doses of 0.005 or 0.02 ml. After 18-24 h, the eyes were examined and the reactions scored. The eye injury was scored as grade 5 (severe irritation) (Hine et al., 1952, 1953).

8.3.2 Sensitization

In a test with 20 "P" strain guinea-pigs, a 5% w/v concentration of "MIX D/D" in corn oil was used and three topical induction applications were followed by a 1% w/v concentration for the topical challenge (method of Buehler, 1965). In 13 out of the 20 guinea-pigs, a positive reaction was obtained. "MIX D/D" has a moderate skin sensitizing potential (Coombs & Carter, 1976a).

8.4 Long-term exposures/carcinogenicity

8.4.1 Oral

8.4.1.1 Rat

Groups of 50 male and 50 female albino rats (age 5 weeks) were fed diets containing nominal concentrations of 0, 10, 30, 100, or 300 mg "MIX D/D"/kg diet for 2 years. Blood samples were collected by suborbital sinus puncture at 3, 6, 12, 18, and 24 months. The "MIX D/D" contained 28.2% *cis*-, 29.0% *trans*-1,3-dichloropropene and 34% 1,2-dichloropropane, without epichlorohydrin.

There were no significant differences throughout the 2-year period between the body weights, food intakes, behaviour, or mortalities of male and female rats fed diets containing "MIX

D/D" and those of control animals. There were no consistent compound-related changes in the haematological parameters.

Statistically significant increases were noted, at 3, 6, and 24 months, in the fasting serum glucose values of rats receiving 300 mg/kg diet and in the serum alkaline phosphatase levels at 12 months compared with controls. These effects were not considered to be biologically significant, because of the size of the response and the lack of a consistent response throughout the study. No other changes were observed in the haematology and clinical chemistry of rats exposed to "MIX D/D" for 2 years.

Urinalyses were performed at 3, 6, 12, 18, and 24 months, and the only statistically significant difference recorded was a lowered specific gravity of urine at 3 months in males receiving 300 mg/kg diet compared with controls. This effect was not correlated with any other changes, and the effect did not occur consistently throughout the study; it was therefore considered to be of doubtful biological significance. No changes attributable to feeding diets containing "MIX D/D" were observed in the organ weights and histopathology at 1 and 2 years (Industr. Biotest Lab., 1978). An audit performed on the study data revealed no major factors that would affect the conclusions of this study. The nominal concentrations of "MIX D/D" specified in the protocol could not be considered representative of the actual concentrations fed to animals. Subsequent work on the volatility of "MIX D/D" in the diet revealed that the average dietary concentrations present at the time of feeding were 40% of the nominal values.

In conclusion, no compound-related effects were observed in rats fed diets containing an average concentration of up to and including 120 mg/kg diet (= nominal concentration of 300 mg/kg diet) "MIX D/D" for two years (Jud et al., 1980a).

8.5 Reproduction, embryotoxicity, and teratogenicity

8.5.1 Reproduction

8.5.1.1 Oral

Charles River CD-strain albino rats (10 males and 20 females) were fed diets containing 0, 10, 30, or 100 mg "MIX D/D" (*cis*-1,3-dichloropropene 28.2%, *trans*-1,3-dichloropropene 29%, 1,2-dichloropropane 34%, without epichlorohydrin) per kg diet in a 3-generation, 2-litter, reproduction study. No statistically significant differences were observed in parental body weights, food consumption, behaviour, or mortalities throughout each 10-week pre-breeding period. Gross pathology, histopathology, and organ weights were similar in all groups. The feeding of diets containing "MIX D/D" did not affect the reproductive performance (mating, fecundity, fertility indices, and parturition incidence) or dam body weights during gestation or post-partum and post-weaning periods. There were no signs of external abnormalities in newborn pups. There were significantly more pups alive at day 1 of lactation in the F_3a litters of the 30 mg/kg group, compared with controls. No differences that were directly related to treatment were noted for survival over a 21-day period, number of pups delivered, or stillbirths. No gross pathological or histopathological differences were observed between treatment and control offspring. Significantly higher mean body weights were recorded at weaning in the F_2b males of the 30 mg/kg group and in males and females of the 100 mg/kg group. Increases were also recorded at weaning in the F_3b generation of 10 mg/kg males and 100 mg/kg females. These increases in mean body weight did not show any consistent relationship with dose or sex and were not considered attributable to "MIX D/D" exposure (Industr. Biotest Lab., 1977a).

An audit of the study data demonstrated that compliance with the protocol was satisfactory and that agreement of the results with more recent data was sufficient to support the conclusions of this study. Subsequent work on the volatility of "MIX D/D" in diet revealed that average concentrations present at the time of feeding were 40% of the nominal values. Thus "MIX D/D" did not produce any effects on the reproductive performance or growth of offspring of rats fed diets containing up to and including 40 mg "MIX D/D"/kg diet (= nominal concentration of 100 mg/kg diet) for 3 generations (40 mg/kg diet, the highest dose level tested is equivalent with 2 mg/kg body weight) (Jud et al., 1980b).

8.5.1.2 Inhalation

In one study (Linnett et al., 1988), groups of 20 male SPF Wistar-derived rats (15 weeks old) and 24 virgin female rats (10 weeks old) were exposed by inhalation to nominal concentrations of 0, 45.4, 136, or 408 mg "MIX D/D"/m^3 (actual concentrations of 0, 64, 145, or 443 mg/m^3 for 6 h/day, 5 days/week, for 10 weeks. The composition of the "MIX D/D" was 28.1% (w/w) *cis*-1,3-dichloropropene, 25.6% *trans*-1,3-dichloropropene, and 25.6% 1,2-dichloropropane and a number of other chlorinated components in percentages up to 5%, but it contained no epichlorohydrin.

Treated males of proven fertility were paired with untreated virgin females at intervals during and after exposure. Groups of 15 treated females were paired with untreated males immediately after the 10-week period. Various aspects of reproduction performance and general toxicity were assessed. Mortality and haematological, clinical-chemical, and urinary parameters were comparable with the controls. Exposure to "MIX D/D" did not produce any adverse effects on the libido, fertility, or morphology of the reproductive tracts of rats of either sex. No treatment-related dominant lethal effects were observed in male rats. Mean body weights of male and female rats at 408 mg/m^3 were significantly decreased. The mean liver and kidney weights were significantly increased in the animals of both sexes exposed to the highest dose level. Histological examination of the organs did not reveal treatment-related changes. This study demonstrates that male and female rats exposed to atmospheres containing up to 443 mg/m^3 "MIX D/D" vapour for 10 weeks did not suffer any impairment of reproductive performance.

8.5.2 Embryotoxicity and teratogenicity

8.5.2.1 Oral

Charles River, albino, female rats received gastric intubations of 0, 30, or 100 mg "MIX D/D"/kg body weight (containing 28% cis-1,3-dichloropropene, 29% trans-1,3-dichloropropene, and 34% 1,2-dichloropropane, without epichlorohydrin) dissolved in corn oil, during days 6 through 15 of pregnancy. The control group was dosed with corn oil. A significant decrease in body weight of the dams receiving 100 mg/kg, compared with the controls, was observed at day 15 of gestation. While no statistically significant reproductive effects occurred, there appears to have been a trend for an increase in the percentage of females with one or more resorption sites. The lack of statistical significance is probably due to the small numbers of animals involved (3 of 17, 6 of 19, and 5 of 15, for the 0, 30, and 100 mg/kg groups, respectively). The maternal toxicity observed in the highest-dose group would account for the apparent increase in resorption sites.

There was a dose-related increase in the incidence of supernumerary ribs (2.8% for controls, 7.6% for the 30 mg/kg group, and 32.3% for the 100 mg/kg per group) and the same was found for the occurrence of non-ossified sternum sections. The incidence of supernumerary ribs over approximately 50 rat teratology studies, in this laboratory, has been within the range 0-26%.

A significant decrease in mean body weight of fetuses from females dosed with 100 mg "MIX D/D"/kg was observed. Maternal toxicity was observed in the 100 mg/kg group, but no malformations, other than supernumerary ribs and non-ossified sternebrae, were observed in this group (Industr. Biotest Lab., 1975).

An audit of the study data demonstrated that there were no major factors to alter the conclusions of this study (O'Sullivan et al., 1980).

8.6 Mutagenicity and related end-points

8.6.1 In vitro studies (microorganisms)

DeLorenzo et al. (1977) tested "MIX D/D" (40% 1,3-dichloropropene and 40% 1,2-dichloropropane) on *Salmonella typhimurium* strains TA98, TA100, TA1535, TA1537, and TA1978, with and without activation. Dose levels of 0, 0.5, 5, 15, and 25 mg/plate were tested. Mutagenic effects were seen with TA100, TA1535, and TA1978, but not with TA98 and TA1537.

Shirasu et al. (1981) studied the mutagenicity of "MIX D/D" in reverse mutation tests using *Salmonella typhimurium* strain TA100, and Moriya et al. (1983) used 5 strains of *Salmonella typhimurium*, TA98, TA100, TA1535, TA1537, and TA1538, and *Escherichia coli* strain WP2 hcr, with and without metabolic activation. "MIX D/D" was tested in dose levels up to 5000 μg/plate. The mutagenic potency in *Salmonella typhimurium* TA100 was 0.0087 revertants/nmole. "MIX D/D" was a direct-acting mutagen in TA100, TA1535, and *E. coli* WP2 hcr, but was not mutagenic in TA1537, TA1538, or TA98.

8.6.2 In vivo studies

Dominant lethality was tested in rats exposed to an atmosphere containing "MIX D/D" vapour for 10 weeks (Linnett et al., 1988, see section 8.5.1.2). No effects on fertility or on implantations were observed even at 443 mg/m^3, the highest concentration tested. This result demonstrates the lack of any significant effects on germ-cell production in rats.

Further evidence of rapid detoxification was found in the negative results of a host-mediated assay using *S. typhimurium*, strain G46, in mice dosed orally with either 60 or 200 mg "MIX D/D"/kg over a 24-h period (Shirasu et al., 1981).

9. EFFECTS ON HUMANS

9.1 General population exposure

A case of acute poisoning occurred a few hours after the accidental ingestion of "MIX D/D". The victim experienced abdominal pain and vomiting. He became semicomatose and exhibited muscle twitching and died (Gosselin et al., 1976; NTP, 1985).

9.2 Occupational exposure

In the period from 1966 to 1971, a total of 13 cases of untoward skin reactions to pesticides were reported in the northern part of the Netherlands. Seven were due to contact with "MIX D/D" caused by inadvertent dripping into the shoes of the applicators during spraying operations. In all cases, acute vesicular dermatitis occurred. Three other cases of dermatitis were described, one being of a contact allergic nature, as confirmed by patch testing, and were diagnosed as orthoergic contact reactions (Nater & Gooskens, 1976).

Nater & Gooskens (1976) and Van Joost & De Jong (1988) described dermatitis in a farmer who had sprayed "MIX D/D" and in a process operator, caused by direct contact. The persons had had previous contact with this substance. Both patients reacted positively in a patch test, with 1% and 0.02% "MIX D/D", respectively.

REFERENCES

Abdalla NA (1974) Distribution, persistence and nematocidal activity of monobromomethane and a pesticide containing 1,3-dichloropropene in soil. Diss Abstr Int, **B35**: 296.

Abdalla NA, Raski DJ, Lear B, & Schmitt RV (1974) Movement, persistence and nematocidal activity of a pesticide containing 1,3-dichloropropene in soils treated for nematode control in replant vineyards. Plant Dis Reptr, **58**: 562-566.

Ahlsdorf B, Stock R, Muller-Wegener U, & Milde G (1989) [The behaviour of selected pesticides in ground water close to the surface in heterogenous loose sediments.] Schriftenr Ver Wasser- Boden- Lufthyg, **79**: 375-385 (in German).

Albrecht WN (1987) Occupational exposure to 1,3-dichloropropene (Telone(R) II) in Hawaiian pineapple culture. Arch Environ Health, **42**(5): 286-291.

Albrecht WN & Chenchin K (1985) Dissipation of 1,2-dibromo-3-chloropropane (DBCP), *cis*-1,3-dichloropropene (1,3-DCP) and dichloropropenes from soil to atmosphere. Bull Environ Contam Toxicol, **34**: 824-831.

Albrecht WN, Hagadone MR, & Chenchin K (1986) Charcoal air sampling tube storage stability and desorption efficiencies of 1,2-dibromo-3-chloropropane (DBCP) and 1,3-dichloropropene (DCP). Bull Environ Contam Toxicol, **36**: 629-634.

Altman J (1969) Effect of chlorinated C_3 hydrocarbons on amino acid production by indigenous soil bacteria. Phytopathology, **59**: 762-766.

Altman J & Lawlor S (1966) The effect of some chlorinated hydrocarbons on certain soil bacteria. J Appl Bacteriol, **29**: 260-265.

Atkins EL, Greywood EA, & MacDonald RL (1973) Toxicity of pesticides and other agricultural chemicals to honey bees. Riverside, California, University of California, Agricultural Extension (Report No. M16 5M Rev. 9/73).

Bakker Y (1968) [Influence of soil decontamination with DD on nitrogen manuring.] Landbouwvoorlichting, **25**(2): 87-88 (in Dutch).

Bartels MJ & Timchalk C (1990) 1,2-Dichloropropane: Investigation of the mechanism of mercapturic acid formation in the rat. Xenobiotica, **20**(10): 1035-1042.

Baruffini A, Cirla AM, Pisati G, Ratti R, & Zedda S (1989) Allergic contact dermatitis from 1,2-dichloropropane. Contact Dermatitis, **20**: 379-380.

Battersby NS (1990a) *Trans*-1,3-dichloropropene: An assessment of ready biodegradability. Internal Report. London, Shell Research Ltd (Unpublished proprietary report SBGR 89.179, submitted to WHO by Shell).

Battersby NS (1990b) An assessment of the inhibitory effect of *cis*- + *trans*-mixture 1,3-dichloropropene on the respiration rate of activated sludge. Internal Report. London, Shell Research Ltd (Unpublished proprietary report SBGR 90.007, submitted to WHO by Shell).

Battersby NS (1990c) An assessment of the inhibitory effect of *cis*-1,3-dichloropropene on the respiration rate of activated sludge. Internal Report. London, Shell Research Ltd (Unpublished proprietary report SBGR 90.005, submitted to WHO by Shell).

Bellomo G & Orrenius S (1985) Altered thiol and calcium homeostasis in oxidative hepatocellular injury. Hepatology, **5**: 876-882.

Belser NO & Castro CE (1971) Biodehalogenation - the metabolism of the nematocides *cis*- and *trans*-3-chloroallyl alcohol by a bacterium isolated from soil. J Agric Food Chem, **19**: 23-26.

Bennett D & Ridge MA (1989) *Trans*-1,3-dichloropropene: Determination of the N-octanol/water partition coefficient using a reverse-phase HPLC method. Internal report. London, Shell Research Ltd (Unpublished proprietary report SBGR 89.133, submitted to WHO by Shell).

Benoit DA, Puglisi FA, & Olson DL (1982) A fathead minnow, *Pimephales promelas*, early life stage toxicity test method evaluation and exposure to four organic chemicals. Environ Pollut, **A28**: 189-197.

Berry DL, Campbell WF, Street JC, & Salunkhe DK (1980) Uptake and metabolism of 1,3-dichloropropene in plants. J Food Saf, 2(4): 247-255.

Beugelink GP (1987) [Chemicals used in soil decontamination heralds of a serious contamination.] H_2O, 20(21): 522-526 (in Dutch).

Blair D (1977) Toxicity of soil fumigants: acute inhalation toxicity of 1,3-dichloropropene. Sittingbourne, Shell Research Ltd, (Unpublished proprietary report TLTR 0002.77, submitted to WHO by Shell).

Bousema MT, Wiemer GR, & Van Joost TH (1991) A classic case of sensitization to DD-95. Contact Dermatitis, **24**: 132-133.

Boyd KW, Emory MB, & Dillon HK (1981) Development of personal sampling and analytical methods for organochlorine compounds. Washington, DC, American Chemical Society, pp 49-64 (ACS Symposium Series No. 149).

Boyland E & Chasseaud LF (1969) The role of glutathione and glutathione-S-transferases in mercapturic acid biosynthesis. Adv Enzymol, **32**: 173-219.

Breslin WJ, Kirk HD, Streeter CM, Quast JF, & Szabo JR (1987) Telone II soil fumigant: Two generation inhalation reproduction study in Fischer 344 rats. (Study No. M003993-015). Midland, Michigan, Dow Chemical Company (Unpublished proprietary report submitted to WHO by Dow Chemical).

Breslin WJ, Kirk HD, Streeter CM, Quast JF, & Szabo JR (1989) 1,3-Dichloropropene: Two generation inhalation reproduction study in Fischer 344 rats. Fundam Appl Toxicol, **12**: 129-143.

Brezis M, Rosen S, Silva P, & Epstein FH (1983) Selective glutathione depletion on function and structure of the isolated perfused rat kidney. Kidney Int, **24**: 178-184.

Bromley S & Cook KA (1981) Evaluation of the soil fumigant, DD, as a nitrification inhibitor. Sittingbourne, Shell Research Ltd (Unpublished proprietary report SBGR 81.295, submitted to WHO by Shell).

Brooks TM, Dean BJ, & Wright AS (1978) Toxicity studies with dichloropropenes; Mutation studies with 1,3-D and *cis*-1,3-dichloropropene and the influence of glutathione on the mutagenicity of *cis*-1,3 dichloropropene in *Salmonella typhimurium*. Sittingbourne, Shell Research Ltd (Unpublished proprietary report TLGR 0081.78, submitted to WHO by Shell).

Brooks TM & Wiggins DE (1989a) Bacterial mutagenicity studies with *trans*-1,3-dichloropropene. Internal report. London, Shell Research Ltd (Unpublished proprietary report SBGR 88.247, submitted to WHO by Shell).

Brooks TM & Wiggins DE (1989b) Genotoxicity studies with *trans*-1,3-dichloropropene: *In vitro* chromosome studies with *trans*-1,3-dichloropropene. Internal report. London, Shell Research Ltd (Unpublished proprietary report SBGR 89.086, submitted to WHO by Shell).

Brooks TM & Wiggins DE (1990) Bacterial mutagenicity studies with *cis*-1,3-dichloropropene. Internal report. London, Shell Research Ltd (Unpublished proprietary report SBGR 89.205, submitted to WHO by Shell).

Brooks TM & Wiggins DE (1991) Genotoxicity studies with *cis*-1,3-dichloropropene: *In vitro* chromosome studies. Internal report. London, Shell Research Ltd (Unpublished proprietary report SBGR 90.049, submitted to WHO by Shell).

Brouwer DH, Brouwer EJ, De Vreede JAF, Van Welie RTH, Vermeulen NPE, & Van Hemmen JJ (1991a) Inhalation exposure to 1,3-dichloropropene in the Dutch flower-bulb culture. Part. I. Environmental monitoring. Arch Environ Contam Toxicol, 20: 1-5.

Brouwer EJ, Evelo CTA, Verplanke AJW, Van Welie RTH, & De Wolff FA (1991b) Biological effect monitoring of occupational exposure to 1,3-dichloropropene: Effects on liver and renal function and on glutathione conjugation. Br J Ind Med, 48: 167-172.

Brown RH & Purnell CJ (1979) Collection and analysis of trace organic vapour pollutants in ambient atmospheres. The performance of a Tenax-GC adsorbent tube. J Chromatogr, 178: 79-90.

Bruckner JV, Mackenzie WF, Ramanathan R, Muralidhara S, Kim HJ, & Dallas CE (1989) Oral toxicity of 1,2-dichloropropane: Acute, short-term and long-term studies in rats. Fundam Appl Toxicol, 12: 713-730.

Buccafusco RJ, Ells SJ, & Leblanc GA (1981) Acute toxicity of priority pollutants to bluegill (*Lepomis macrochirus*). Bull Environ Contam Toxicol, 26: 446-452.

Buehler EV (1965) Delayed contact hypersensitivity in the guinea-pig. Arch Dermatol, 91: 171-177.

California State Water Resources Control Board (1983) 1,2-Dichloropropene (1,2-D) and 1,3-dichloropropene (1,3-D). California State Water Resources Control Board, Toxic Substances Control Programme (Unpublished special project draft report).

Carere A & Morpurgo G (1981) Comparison of the mutagenic activity of pesticides *in vitro* in various short-term assays. In: Kappas A ed. Progress in environmental mutagenesis and carcinogenesis. Amsterdam, Oxford, New York, Elsevier Science Publishers, pp 87-104 (Progress in Mutation Research, Volume 2).

Carter B (1975) Toxicity of soil fumigants: acute oral toxicity of D-D to mice and dogs. Sittingbourne, Shell Research Ltd (Unpublished proprietary report TLGR 0034.75, submitted to WHO by Shell).

Casini AF, Maellaro E, Pompella A, Ferrali M, & Comporti M (1987) Lipid peroxidation, protein thiols and calcium homeostasis in bromobenzene-induced liver damage. Biochem Pharmacol, 36: 3689-3695.

Castro CE & Belser NO (1966) Hydrolysis of *cis*- and *trans*-1,3-dichloropropene in wet soil. J Agric Food Chem, 14(1): 69-70.

Clark DG (1980) D-D: A 10-week inhalation study of mating behaviour, fertility and toxicity in male and female rats. Sittingbourne, Shell Research Ltd (Unpublished proprietary report TLGR 80.023, submitted to WHO by Shell).

Climie IJG, Hutson DH, Morrison BJ, & Stoydin G (1979) Glutathione conjugation in the detoxication of (Z)-1-3-dichloropropene (a component of the nematocide D-D) in the rat. Xenobiotica, 9(3): 149-156.

Coate WB & Voelker RW (1979b) Final report: 90-day inhalation toxicity study in rats and mice. Telone II. Vienna, Virginia, Hazleton Laboratories America Inc. (Unpublished proprietary report submitted to WHO by Dow Chemical).

Coate WB & Voelker RW (1979a) Addendum to final report: 90-day inhalation toxicity study in rats and mice. Telone II. Vienna, Virginia, Hazleton Laboratories America Inc. (Unpublished proprietary report submitted to WHO by Dow Chemical).

Collins CJ (1989) *Trans*-1,3-dichloropropene: Acute inhalation toxicity study - LC_{50} rats (4-hour exposure). Harrogate, United Kingdom, Hazleton Laboratories (Unpublished proprietary report submitted to WHO by Shell).

Connors TF, Stuart JD, & Cope JB (1990) Chromatographic and mutagenic analyses of 1,2-dichloropropane and 1,3-dichloropropylene and their degradation products. Bull Environ Contam Toxicol, 44: 288-293.

Coombs AD & Carter BI (1976a) The toxicity of soil fumigants: Acute toxicity, skin irritation and skin sensitizing potential of current product D-D. Sittingbourne, Shell Research Ltd (Unpublished proprietary report TLTR 0021.76, submitted to WHO by Shell).

Coombs AD & Carter BI (1976b) The toxicity of soil fumigants: Acute toxicity, skin irritation and skin sensitizing potential of 1,3-dichloropropene (95% w/w a.m.). Sittingbourne, Shell Research Ltd (Unpublished proprietary report TLTR 0023.76, submitted to WHO by Shell).

Cotruvo JA (1985) Organic micropollutants in drinking water: An overview. Sci Total Environ, 47: 7-26.

Cracknell S, Jackson GC, & Hardy CJ (1987) Telone II (1,3-dichloropropene): acute inhalation study in rats. 4-hour exposure. Huntingdon, United Kingdom, Huntingdon Research Centre Ltd (Prepared for Dow Chemical Europe, Horgen, Switzerland) (Unpublished proprietary report submitted to WHO by Dow Chemical Company).

Crebelli R, Conti G, Conti L, & Carere A (1984) Induction of somatic segregation by halogenated aliphatic hydrocarbons in *Aspergillus nidulans*. Mutat Res, **138**: 33-38.

Creedy CL (1983) The modulation of the bacterial mutagenicity of the (Z)- and (E)-isomers of 1,3-dichloropropene by glutathione and subcellular fractions from rat liver. Sittingbourne, Shell Research Ltd (Unpublished proprietary report SBGR 83.380, submitted to WHO by Shell).

Creedy CL & Hutson DH (1982) The bacterial mutagenicity of (E)-1,3-dichloropropene and its modulation by glutathione. Sittingbourne, Shell Research Ltd (Unpublished proprietary report SBGR 82.335, submitted to WHO by Shell).

Creedy CL, Brooks TM, Dean BJ, Hutson DH, & Wright AS (1984) The protective action of glutathione on the microbial mutagenicity of the Z- and E-isomers of 1,3-dichloropropene. Chem-Biol Interact, **50**(1): 39-48.

Daft JL (1989) Determination of fumigants and related chemicals in fatty and non-fatty foods. J Agric Food Chem, **37**: 560-564.

Dawson GW, Jennings AL, Drozdowski D, & Rider E (1977) The acute toxicity of 47 industrial chemicals to fresh and salt water fishes. J Hazard Mater, **1**: 303-318.

De Lorenzo F, Degl'Innocenti S, Ruocco A, Silengo L, & Cortese R (1977) Mutagenicity of pesticides containing 1,3-dichloropropene. Cancer Res, **37**: 1915-1917.

Dietz FK, Dittenber DA, & Kastl PE (1982) 1,3-Dichloropropene: Effects on tissue non-protein sulfhydryl content and blood concentration time profile, probe study. Internal report. Midland, Michigan, Dow Chemical Company (Unpublished proprietary report submitted to WHO by Dow Chemical).

Dietz FK, Hermann EA, & Ramsey JC (1984a) The pharmacokinetics of ^{14}C-1,3-dichloropropene in rats and mice following oral administration. (Presented as poster No. 585 at 23rd Annual Society of Toxicology Conference, Atlanta, Georgia, 15 March 1984). Toxicologist, **4**: 147 (Abstract 585).

Dietz FK, Dittenber DA, Kirk HD, & Ramsey JC (1984b) Non-protein sulfhydryl content and macro-molecular binding in rats and mice following oral administration of 1,3-dichloropropene. (Presented as poster No. 586 at 23rd Annual Society of Toxicology Conference, Atlanta, Georgia, 15 March 1984). Toxicologist, **4**(1): 147 (Abstract 586).

Dietz FK, Hermann EA, Kastl PE, Dittenber DA, & Ramsey JC (1985) 1,3-Dichloropropene: Pharmacokinetics, effect on tissue non-protein sulfhydryls, and macromolecular binding in Fischer 344 rats and $B_6C_3F_1$ mice following oral administration. Freeport, Texas, Dow Chemical Company USA (Unpublished proprietary report HET: K-6409-11, submitted to WHO by Dow Chemical).

Dilling WL, Tefertiller NB, & Kallos GJ (1975) Evaporation rates and reactivities of methylene chloride, chloroform, 1.1.1-trichloroethane, trichloroethylene, tetrachloroethylene and other chlorinated compounds in dilute aqueous solutions. Environ Sci Technol, **9**(9): 833-838.

Di Nucci A, Imbriani M, Ghittori S, Gregotti C, Baldi C, Locatelli C, Manzo L, & Capodaglio E (1988) 1,2-Dichloropropane-induced liver toxicity. Clinical data and preliminary studies in rats. The target organ and the toxic process. Arch Toxicol, **12**(Suppl): 370-374.

Dipaolo JA & Doniger J (1982) Neoplastic transformation of Syrian hamster cells by putative epoxide metabolites of commercially utilized chloroalkenes. J Natl Cancer Inst, **69**(2): 531-534.

Dommergues Y (1959) Influence des nématocides sur l'activité biologique du sol. Fruits (Paris), **14**(4): 177-181.

Dowty B, Carlisle D, & Laseter JL (1975) Halogenated hydrocarbons in New Orleans drinking water and blood plasma. Science, **187**: 75-77.

Draize JH, Woodard G, & Calvery HO (1944) Methods for the study of irritation and toxicity of substances applied topically to the skin and mucous membranes. J Pharmacol Exp Ther, **82**: 377-390.

Dubey HD, Riera A, & Rodriguez RL (1975) Effects of the nematocides Nemagon and DD on mineralization, nitrification, soil microbial population, and soil fertility status of two tropical soils. J Agric Univ Puerto Rico, **59**(1): 43-50.

Dynamic Corporation (1991) Herd profile: 1,2-Dichloropropane. CAS No. 78-87-5 (Draft). Washington, DC, US Environmental Protection Agency, Health and Environmental Review Division, 12 pp.

Eadsforth CV (1987) Biological monitoring of operators for exposure to D-D during filling operations in CFD loods 2, SNR/C Pernis during 1985-86. Internal report. Rotterdam, Shell Research Ltd, Pernis Biomedical Laboratory (Unpublished proprietary report submitted to WHO by Shell).

Eadsforth CV, Rocchi PSJ, & Tuinman CP (1987) A monitoring study of the exposure to 1,3-dichloropropene during a single application in Germany of Shell D-D 92 nematocide. Internal report. The Hague, Shell Research Ltd, Safety and Environmental Division (Unpublished proprietary report submitted to WHO by Shell).

Edmiston S & Maddy KT (1987) Summary of illness and injuries reported in California by physicians in 1986 as potentially related to pesticides. Vet Hum Toxicol, **29**(5): 391-397.

Edwards CA & Lofty JR (1969) The influence of agricultural practice on soil micro-arthropod populations. Syst Assoc Publ, **8**: 237-247.

Edwards CA (1983) Development of a standardized laboratory method for assessing the toxicity of chemical substances to earthworms. Brussels, Commission of the European Community (Report EUR 8714 EN).

Eichelberger JW, Bellar TA, Donnelly JP, & Budde WL (1990) Determination of volatile organics in drinking water with USEPA method 524.2 and the ion trap detector. J Chromatogr Sci, **28**: 460-467.

Elgar KE, Hughes DG, & Reiff B (1965) Residues of DD in samples of water from France (Technical Memorandum 55/65). Sittingbourne, Woodstock Agricultural Research Centre, Technical Service Laboratory (Unpublished proprietary data submitted to WHO by Shell).

Elliot JM, Marks CF, & Tu CM (1972) Effects of nematicides on *Pratylenchus penetrans*, soil microflora, and flue-cured tobacco. Can J Plant Sci, **52**(1): 1-11.

Elliot JM, Marks CF, & Tu CM (1974) Effects of the nematicides DD and Mocap on soil nitrogen, soil microflora, populations of *Pratylenchus penetrans*, and flue-cured tobacco. Can J Plant Sci, **54**: 801-809.

Elliot JM, Marks CF, & Tu CM (1977) Effects of certain nematicides on soil nitrogen, soil nitrifiers, and populations of *Pratylenchus penetrans* in flue-cured tobacco. Can J Plant Sci, **57**: 143-154.

Ennik GC, Kort J, & Luesink B (1964) The influence of soil disinfection with DD, certain components of DD and some other compounds with nematocidal activity on the growth of white clover. Neth J Plant Pathol, **70**: 117-135.

Fishbein L (1979) Potential halogenated industrial carcinogenic and mutagenic chemicals. Sci Total Environ, **11**: 223-257.

Fisher GD & Kilgore WW (1988a) Mercapturic acid excretion by rats following inhalation exposure to 1,3-dichloropropene. Fundam Appl Toxicol, **11**: 300-307.

Fisher GD & Kilgore WW (1988b) Tissue levels of glutathione following acute inhalation of 1,3-dichloropropene. J Toxicol Environ Health, **2**: 171-182.

Fisher GD & Kilgore WW (1989) Pharmacokinetics of S-[3-chloroprop-2-enyl]-glutathione in rats following acute inhalation exposure to 1,3-dichloropropene. Xenobiotica, **19**(3): 269-278.

Flessel P, Goldsmith JR, Kahn E, & Wesolowski JJ (1978) Acute and possible long-term effects of 1,3-dichloropropene-California. Morb Mortal Wkly Rep, **271**: 50, 55.

Fong HR & Maykoski R (1985) Air exposure monitoring of EHAP personnel during a Telone II soil translocation study in Fresno County. Sacramento, California, California Department of Food and Agriculture, Division of Pest Management, Environmental Protection and Worker Safety, Worker Health and Safety Unit, 6 pp (Unpublished report HS-1299).

Galloway SM, Armstrong MJ, Reuben C, Colman S, Brown B, Cannon C, Bloom AD, Nakamura F, Ahmed M, Duk S, Rimpo J, Margolin BB, Resnick MA, Anderson B, & Zieger E (1987) Chromosome aberrations and sister chromatid exchanges in Chinese hamster ovary cells: Evaluation of 108 chemicals. Environ Mol Mutagen, **10**(Suppl): 1-175.

Gardner JR (1989a) DD-95 (*cis-* + *trans*-mixture 1,3-dichloropropene): Acute oral toxicity. Internal report. London, Shell Research Ltd (Unpublished proprietary report SBGR 89.005, submitted to WHO by Shell).

Gardner JR (1989b) *Cis*-1,3-dichloropropene: Acute oral and dermal toxicity, skin and eye irritancy and skin sensitisation potential. Internal report. London, Shell Research Ltd (Unpublished proprietary report SBGR 89.007, submitted to WHO by Shell).

Gardner JR (1989c) *Trans*-1,3-dichloropropene: Acute oral and dermal toxicity, skin and eye irritancy and skin sensitising potential. Internal report. London, Shell Research Ltd (Unpublished proprietary report SBGR 88.286, submitted to WHO by Shell).

Girling AE (1989a) *Cis*-1,3-dichloropropene: Acute toxicity to *Salmo gairdneri, Daphnia magna* and *Selenastrum capricornutum*. London, Shell Research Ltd (Unpublished proprietary report SBGR 89.118, submitted to WHO by Shell).

Girling AE (1989b) *Cis + trans*-1,3-dichloropropene: Acute toxicity to *Salmo gairdneri, Daphnia magna* and *Selenastrum capricornutum*. London, Shell Research Ltd (Unpublished proprietary report SBGR 89.159, submitted to WHO by Shell).

Girling AE (1989c) *Trans*-1,3-dichloropropene: Acute toxicity to *Salmo gairdneri, Daphnia magna* and *Selenastrum capricornutum*. London, Shell Research Ltd (Unpublished proprietary report SBGR 89.160, submitted to WHO by Shell).

Goffart H & Heiling A (1958) [Side effects of nematode control with Shell D-D and related agents.] Nematologica, 3: 213-228 (in German with English summary).

Gollapudi BB, Bruce RJ, & Hinze CA (1985) Evaluation of Telone II soil fumigant in the mouse bone marrow micronucleus test. Freeport, Texas, Dow Chemical Company USA (Unpublished proprietary report submitted to WHO by Dow Chemical).

Gorzinski SJ & Johnson KA (1989) Neurotoxicologic examination of Fischer 344 rats exposed to 1,2-dichloropropane (DCP) via gavage for 2 weeks. Internal report. Midland, Michigan, Dow Chemical Company (Unpublished proprietary report submitted to WHO by Dow Chemical).

Gosselin R, Hodge H, Smith R, & Gleason M (1976) Clinical toxicology of commercial products, 4th ed. Baltimore, Maryland, Williams and Wilkins Co., pp 119-121.

Greve PA, Klapwijk SP, & Linders JBHJ (1989) [Pesticides in surface water in the bulb-growing area near Langeveld.] Bilthoven, The Netherlands, National Institute of Public Health and Environmental Protection (Unpublished report No. 638812001) (in Dutch).

Grzywa Z & Rudzki E (1981) Dermatitis from dichloropropene. Contact Dermatitis, 7: 151-152.

Haemisegger ER, Jones AD, & Reinhardt FL (1985) EPA's experience with assessment of site-specific environmental problems: A review of IEMD's geographic study of Philadelphia. (Prepared for presentations at the 78th Annual Meeting of the Air Pollution Control Association, Detroit, Michigan, 16-21 June 1985). Washington, DC, US Environmental Protection Agency, pp 1-20 (Report 85-63-6).

Hallberg GR (1989) Pesticide pollution of groundwater in the humid United States. Agric Ecosyst Environ, 26: 299-367.

Hanley TR Jr, John-Greene JA, Young JT, Calhoun LL, & Rao KS (1987) Evaluation of the effects of inhalation exposure to 1,3-dichloropropene on fetal development in rats and rabbits. Fundam Appl Toxicol, 8: 562-570.

Hanley TR Jr, Berdasco NM, Battjes JE, & Johnson KA (1989a) Propylene dichloride: Oral teratology study in New Zealand white rabbits. Internal report. Midland, Michigan, Dow Chemical Company (Unpublished proprietary report submitted to WHO by Dow Chemical).

Hanley TR Jr, Kirk HD, Bond DM, Firchau HM, & Johnson KA (1989b) Propylene dichloride: Dominant lethal study in Sprague-Dawley rats. Internal report. Midland, Michigan, Dow Chemical Company (Unpublished proprietary report submitted to WHO by Dow Chemical).

Hanley TR Jr, Kirk HD, Berdasco NM, & Johnson KA (1990) Evaluation of the developmental toxicity of propylene dichloride in rats and rabbits. Teratology, 41(5): 562 (Abstract P54).

Haseman JK, Crawford DD, Huff JE, Boorman GA, & McConnell EE (1984) Results from 86 two-year carcinogenicity studies conducted by the national toxicology program. J Toxicol Environ Health, 14: 621-639.

Haworth S, Lawlor T, Mortelmans K, Speck W, & Zeiger E (1983) *Salmonella* mutagenicity test results for 250 chemicals. Environ. Mutagen, 1(Suppl): 3-142.

Hayes WJ Jr (1982) Pesticides studied in man. Baltimore, Maryland, Williams and Wilkins Co., pp 162, 163.

Hazleton Laboratories America, Inc. (1979) Subacute inhalation toxicity study of D-D soil fumigant in CD-1 mice and albino Fischer 344 rats. Vienna, Virginia, Hazleton Laboratories America Inc. (Prepared for Shell Oil Company, Houston, Texas) (Unpublished proprietary report No. 776-132, submitted to WHO by Shell).

Heitmuller PT, Hollister TA, & Parrish PR (1981) Acute toxicity of 54 industrial chemicals to sheephead minnows (*Cyprinodon variegatus*). Bull Environ Contam Toxicol, 27: 596-604.

Heppel LA, Highman B, & Porterfield VT (1946) Toxicology of 1,2-dichloropropane (propylene dichloride). II Influence of dietary factors on the toxicity of dichloropropane. J Pharmacol Exp Ther, 87: 11-17.

Hermann BW & Matsuyama H (1982) Freezer storage stability of D-D soil fumigant: Shell Development Company's monthly research summary (July 1982). Modesto, California, Shell Development Company (Unpublished proprietary report submitted to WHO by Shell).

Heungens A & Van Daele E (1974) Evolution of the soil fauna in Begonia culture by repeated applications of dichloropropane-dichloropropene. Agric Environ, 1: 251-258.

Hiatt MH (1983) Determination of volatile organic compounds in fish samples by vacuum distillation and fused silica capillary gas chromatography/mass spectrometry. Anal Chem, 55: 506-516.

Hine CH, Anderson HH, Kodama JK, Morse M, & McDaniel HC (1952) Studies on the toxicity of CBP-55 and D-D. San Francisco, University of California, School of Medicine, Division of Pharmacology and Experimental Therapeutics (Prepared for Shell Development Company, California) (Unpublished proprietary report No. U.C. 184, submitted to WHO by Shell).

Hine CH, Anderson HH, Moon HD, Kodama JK, Morse M, & Jacobsen NW (1953) Toxicology and safe handling of CBP-55 (Technical 1-Chloro-3-bromopropene-1). Arch Ind Hyg Occup Med, 7: 118-136.

Hoogsteen KJ (1986) [Micro pollution in 3 water-winning areas.] H_2O, 19(3): 48-52 (in Dutch).

HSE (1990) Chlorinated hydrocarbon solvent vapours in air. Methods for the determination of hazardous substances (MDHS 28). London, Health and Safety Executive, Occupational Medicine and Hygiene Laboratory, pp. 1-7.

Hutson DH (1984) The role of oxidation in the bacterial mutagenicity of (Z)-1,3-dichloropropene. Sittingbourne, Shell Research Ltd (Unpublished proprietary report SBGR 83.049, submitted to WHO by Shell).

Hutson DH & Stoydin G (1977) The reaction of D-D components with glutathione. Sittingbourne, Shell Research Ltd (Unpublished proprietary report TLGR 0041-77, submitted to WHO by Shell).

Hutson DH, Moss JA, & Pickering BA (1971) The excretion and retention of components of the soil fumigant D-D, and their metabolites in the rat. Food Cosmet Toxicol, 9(5): 677-680.

IARC (1986) Some halogenated hydrocarbons and pesticide exposures. Lyon, International Agency for Research on Cancer, pp 113-130, 131-147 (IARC Monographs on the Evaluation of the Carcinogenic Risk of Chemicals to Humans, Volume 41).

IARC (1987) Overall evaluations of carcinogenicity: An updating of IARC monographs, Volumes 1 to 42. Lyon, International Agency for Research on Cancer, pp 195-196 (IARC Monographs on the Evaluation of Carcinogenic Risks to Humans, Supplement 7).

Imberti R, Calabrese SR, Emilio G, Marchi L, & Giuffrida L (1987) [Acute solvent poisoning: aliphatic chlorinated hydrocarbons.] Min Anest, 53: 399-403 (in Italian).

Imberti R, Mapelli A, Colombo P, Richelmi P, Berte F, & Bellomo G (1990) 1,2-Dichloropropane (DCP) toxicity is correlated with DCP-induced glutathione (GSH) depletion and is modulated by factors affecting intracellular GSH. Arch Toxicol, 64: 459-465.

Industrial Biotest Laboratories Inc. (1972) Primary skin irritation tests with three samples in albino rabbits. Northbrook, Illinois, Industrial Biotest Laboratories Inc. (Unpublished proprietary report No. IBT A.2484, submitted to WHO by Shell).

Industrial Biotest Laboratories Inc. (1975) Teratogenic study with D-D in albino rats. Northbrook, Illinois, Industrial Biotest Laboratories Inc. (Prepared for Shell Kagaku Kabushiki Kaisha) (Unpublished proprietary report No. IBT 623-06212, submitted to WHO by Shell).

Industrial Biotest Laboratories Inc. (1977a) Three generation reproduction study with D-D in albino rats. Northbrook, Illinois, Industrial Biotest Laboratories Inc. (Prepared for Shell Kagaku Kabushiki Kaisha) (Unpublished proprietary report No. IBT 621-06002, submitted to WHO by Shell).

Industrial Biotest Laboratories Inc. (1977b) Two year chronic and toxicity study with D-D compound in beagle dogs. Northbrook, Illinois, Industrial Biotest Laboratories Inc. (Prepared for Shell Kagaku Kabushiki Kaisha) (Unpublished proprietary report No. IBT 651-06000, submitted to WHO by Shell).

Industrial Biotest Laboratories Inc. (1978) Two year chronic and toxicity study with D-D in albino rats. Northbrook, Illinois, Industrial Biotest Laboratories Inc. (Prepared for Shell Kagaku Kabushiki Kaisha) (Unpublished proprietary report No. IBT 621-06001, submitted to WHO by Shell).

Jeffrey MM (1987a) Telone II soil fumigant: Primary dermal irritation study in New Zealand White rabbits. Midland, Michigan, Dow Chemical Company (Unpublished proprietary report No. M-003993-017B, submitted to WHO by Dow Chemical).

Jeffrey MM (1987b) Telone II soil fumigant: Primary eye irritation study in New Zealand White rabbits. Midland, Michigan, Dow Chemical Company (Unpublished proprietary report No. M-003993-017C, submitted to WHO by Dow Chemical).

Jeffrey MM (1987c) Telone II soil fumigant: Dermal sensitization potential in the Hartley albino guinea-pig. Midland, Michigan, Dow Chemical Company (Unpublished proprietary report No. DR-003993-017E, submitted to WHO by Dow Chemical).

Jeffrey MM, Battjer JE, & Lomax LG (1987) Telone II soil fumigant. Acute oral toxicity study in Fischer 344 rats. Internal report. Midland, Michigan, Dow Chemical Company (Unpublished proprietary report submitted to WHO by Dow Chemical).

John JA, Kloes PM, Calhoun LL, & Young JT (1983) Technical grade 1,3-dichloropropene: Inhalation teratology study in Fischer 344 rats and New Zealand White rabbits. Internal report. Midland, Michigan, Dow Chemical Company (Unpublished proprietary report submitted to WHO by Dow Chemical).

Johnson KA & Gorzinski SJ (1988) Neurotoxicologic examination of rats exposed to 1,2-dichloropropane (DCP) via gavage for 13 weeks. Internal report. Midland, Michigan, Dow Chemical Company (Unpublished proprietary report submitted to WHO by Dow Chemical).

Jones AR & Gibson J (1980) 1,2-dichloropropane: metabolism and fate in the rat. Xenobiotica, 10(11): 835-846.

Jones JR & Collier TA (1986a) Telone II: OECD 401 Acute oral toxicity test in the rat (Project No. 44/83). Horgen, Switzerland, Dow Chemical Europe S.A. (Unpublished proprietary report submitted to WHO by Dow Chemical).

Jones JR & Collier TA (1986b) Telone II: OECD 402 Acute dermal toxicity test in the rat (Project No. 44/84). Horgen, Switzerland, Dow Chemical Europe S.A. (Unpublished proprietary report submitted to WHO by Dow Chemical).

Jud VA, Kincke VL, O'Sullivan PK, Schweizer AD, & Parker CM (1980a) Audit of Industrial Bio-Test Laboratories Study No. 621-06001: Two year chronic oral toxicity study with D-D in albino rats (Regulatory Information Record No. WRC RIR-5). Houston, Texas, Shell Development Company (Unpublished proprietary report submitted to WHO by Shell).

Jud VA, Kincke VL, Schweizer AD, & Lu CC (1980b) Audit of Industrial Bio-Test Laboratories Study No. 621-06002: Three generation reproduction study with D-D in albino rats (Regulatory Information Record No. WRC RIR-7). Houston, Texas, Shell Development Company (Unpublished proprietary report submitted to WHO by Shell).

Kämpfe K (1973) [Results of the combined application of anhydrous ammonia and a mixture of dichloropropane and dichloropropene (DD) as a nitrification inhibitor in autumn.] Arch Acker-Pflanzenbau Bodenkd, 17(10): 827-835 (in German).

Kastl PE & Hermann EA (1983) Determination of *cis*- and *trans*-1,3-dichloropropene in whole rat blood by gas chromatography and gas chromatography-chemical ionization mass spectrometry with selected ion monitoring. J Chromatogr, 265: 277-283.

Kenaga EE (1980) Predicted bioconcentration factors and soil sorption coefficients of pesticides and other chemicals. Ecotoxicol Environ Saf, 4: 26-38.

Kier LE, Brusick DJ, Auletta AE, Von Halle ES, Brown MM, Simmon VF, Dunkel V, McCann J, Mortelmans K, Prival M, Rao TK, & Ray V (1986) The *Salmonella typhimurium*/mammalian microsomal assay. A report of the US Environmental Protection Agency gene-Tox program. Mutat Res, 16: 69-240.

Kirk HD, Hanley TR Jr, Johnson KA, & Dietz FK (1989) Propylene dichloride: Oral teratology study in Sprague-Dawley rats. Internal report. Midland, Michigan, Dow Chemical Company (Unpublished proprietary report submitted to WHO by Dow Chemical).

Kirk HD, Hanley TR Jr, Bond DM, Firchau HM, Peck CN, Stebbins KE, & Johnson KA (1990) Propylene dichloride: Two-generation reproduction study in Sprague-Dawley rats. Internal report. Midland, Michigan, Dow Chemical Company (Unpublished proprietary report submitted to WHO by Dow Chemical).

Kline SA, McCoy EC, Rosenkranz HS, & Van Duuren BL (1982) Mutagenicity of chloroalkene epoxides in bacterial systems. Mutat Res, 101: 115-125.

Kloes PM, Calhoun LL, Young JT, & John JA (1983) Telone II: Inhalation teratology probe study in Fischer 344 rats and New Zealand White rabbits. Internal report. Midland, Michigan, Dow Chemical Company (Unpublished proprietary report submitted to WHO by Dow Chemical).

Könemann H (1981) Quantitative structure-activity relationships in fish toxicity studies. Toxicology, 19: 209-221.

Krijgsheld KR & Van der Gen A (1986) Assessment of the impact of the emission of certain organochlorine compounds on the aquatic environment. Part II: Allylchloride, 1,3- and 2,3-dichloropropene. Chemosphere, 15(7): 861-880.

Lagas P, Verdam B, & Loch JPG (1989) Threat to groundwater quality by pesticides in the Netherlands. In: Groundwater management: Quantity and quality. Proceedings of the Benidorm Symposium, October 1989, pp 171-180 (IAHS Publication No. 188).

Larcan A, Lambert H, Laprevote MC, & Gustin B (1977) Acute poisoning induced by dichloropropane. Acta Pharmacol Toxicol, 41: 330.

Lebbink G & Kolenbrander GJ (1974) Quantitative effect of fumigation with 1,3-dichloropropene mixtures and with metham sodium on the soil nitrogen status. Agric Environ, 1: 283-292.

Lebbink G, Proper B, & Nipshagen A (1989) Accelerated degradation of 1,3-dichloropropene. Acta Hortic, 255: 361-371.

Leblanc GA (1980) Acute toxicity of priority pollutants to water flea (*Daphnia magna*). Bull Environ Contam Toxicol, 24: 684-691.

Leblanc GA (1984) Interspecies relationships in acute toxicity of chemicals to aquatic organisms. Environ Toxicol Chem, 3: 47-60.

Leiber MA & Berk HC (1984) Development and validation of an air monitoring method for 1,3-dichloropropene, *trans*-1,2,3-trichloropropene *cis*-1,2,3-trichloropropene 1,1,2,3-tetrachloropropene, 2,3,3-trichloro-2-propen-1-ol and 1,1,2,2,3-pentachloropropane. Anal Chem, 56: 2134-2137.

Leistra M (1970) Distribution of 1,3-dichloropropene over the phases in soil. J Agric Food Chem, 18(6): 1124-1126.

Leistra M & Boesten JJTI (1989) Pesticide contamination of groundwater in Western Europe. Agric Ecosyst Environ, 26: 369-389.

Leistra M, Groen AE, Crum SJH, & Van der Pas LJT (1991) Transformation rate of 1,3-dichloropropene and 3-chloroallyl alcohol in topsoil and subsoil material of flower-bulb fields. Pestic Sci, 31: 197-207.

Li M (1979) A systems approach to controlling pesticides in the San Joaquin Valley, Ecosystem studies of the National Science Foundation, University of California, Davis.

Ligocki MP, Leuenberger C, & Pankow JG (1985) Trace organic compounds in rain - II. Gas scavenging of neutral organic compounds. Atmos Environ, 19(10): 1609-1617.

Linnett SL, Clark DG, Blair D, & Cassidy SL (1988) Effects of subchronic inhalation of D-D (1,3-dichloropropene/1,2-dichloropropane) on reproduction in male and female rats. Fundam Appl Toxicol, 10: 214-223.

Loch JPG & Verdam B (1989) Pesticide residues in groundwater in the Netherlands: State of observations and future directions of research. Schriftenr Ver Wasser- Boden- Lufthyg, 79: 349-363.

Lomax LG, Calhoun LL, Stott WT, & Franson LE (1987) Telone II soil fumigant: 2-year inhalation chronic toxicity-oncogenicity study in rats (Study No. M 003993-009R). Midland, Michigan, Dow Chemical Company (Unpublished proprietary report submitted to WHO by Dow Chemical).

Lomax LG, Stott WT, Johnson KA, Calhoun LL, Yano BL, & Quast JF (1989) The chronic toxicity and oncogenicity of inhaled technical-grade 1,3-dichloropropene in rats and mice. Fundam Appl Toxicol, 12: 418-431.

Loveday KS, Lugo MH, Resnick MA, Anderson BE, & Zeiger E (1989) Chromosome aberration and sister chromatid exchange tests in Chinese hamster ovary cells *in vitro*: II. Results with 20 chemicals. Environ Mol Mutagen, 13: 60-94.

McCall PJ (1987) Hydrolysis of 1,3-dichloropropene in dilute aqueous solution. Pestic Sci, 19: 235-242.

McKenry MV & Thomason IJ (1974) Dosage values obtained following pre-plant fumigation for perennials. I 1,3-dichloropropene nematicides in eleven field situations. Pestic Sci, 7: 521-534.

Maddy KT, Fong HR, Lowe JA, Conrad DW, & Fredrickson AS (1982) A study of well water in selected Californian communities for residues of 1,3-dichloropropene, chloroallyl alcohol and 49 organophosphate or chlorinated hydrocarbon pesticides. Bull Environ Contam Toxicol, 29: 354-359.

Maddy KT, Edmiston S, & Richmond D (1990) Illness, injuries, and deaths from pesticide exposures in California 1949-1988. Rev Environ Contam Toxicol, 114: 58-99.

Markovitz A & Crosby WH (1984) Chemical carcinogenesis: A soil fumigant, 1,3-dichloropropene as possible cause of hematologic malignancies. Arch Intern Med, 144: 1409-1411.

Matsui S, Yamamoto R, & Yamada H (1989) The Bacillus subtilis/microsome REC-assay for the detection of DNA damaging substances which may occur in chlorinated and ozonated waters. Water Sci Technol, 21: 875-887.

Mayer FL & Ellersieck MR (1986) Manual of acute toxicity: Interpretation and data base for 410 chemicals and 66 species of freshwater animals. Washington, DC, US Department of the Interior, Fish and Wildlife Service, pp 506-553 (Resource Publication No. 160).

Mehta BV, Patel GJ, & Dangarwala RT (1963) Effects of fumigation and other measures for nematode control on the production of nitrate in *Goradu* soil. J Indian Soc Soil Sci, 11: 361-371.

Mendrala AL (1985) Evaluation of Telone II in the rat hepatocyte unscheduled DNA synthesis assay. Midland, Michigan, Dow Chemical Company (Unpublished proprietary report submitted to WHO by Dow Chemical).

Mendrala AL (1986) The evaluation of Telone II soil fumigant in the Chinese hamster ovary cell/hypoxanthine (guanine) phosphoribosyl transferase (CHO/HGPRT) forward mutation assay. Midland, Michigan, Dow Chemical Company (Unpublished proprietary report submitted to WHO by Dow Chemical).

Meyer AL (1980) Mutagenicity studies with *cis*-1,3-dichloropropene in cultured mammalian cells. Sittingbourne, Shell Research Ltd (Unpublished proprietary report TLGR 80.022, submitted to WHO by Shell).

Mitchell JR, Jollow DJ, Potter WZ, Gilette JR, & Brodie BB (1973) Acetaminophen induced hepatic damage. IV. Protective role of glutathione. J Pharmacol Exp Ther, **1877**: 211-217.

Miyaoka T, Yamashita E, Hasegawa T, Akiyama M, Tsuda S, & Shirasu Y (1990) Mechanism of 1,3-dichloropropene-induced hepatotoxicity in mice. J Pestic Sci, **15**: 419-425.

Moje W, Martin JP, & Baines RC (1957) Structural effects of some organic compounds on soil organisms and citrus seedlings grown in an old citrus soil. J Agric Food Chem, 5(10): 32-36.

Moriya M, Ohta T, Watanabe K, Miyazawa T, Kato K, & Shirasu Y (1983) Further mutagenicity studies on pesticides in bacterial reversion assay systems. Mutat Res, **116**: 185-216.

Munnecke DE & Van Gundy SD (1979) Movement of fumigants in soil, dosage responses, and differential effects. Annu Rev Phytopathol, 17: 405-429.

Nater JP & Gooskens VHJ (1976) Occupational dermatosis due to a soil fumigant. Contact Dermatitis, **2**: 227-229.

Neudecker T & Henschler D (1986) Mutagenicity of chloro-olefins in the Salmonella/mammalian microsome test. III. Metabolic activation of the allylic chloropropenes allylchloride, 1,3-dichloropropene, 2,3-dichloro-1-propene, 1,2,3-trichloropropene, 1,1,2,3-tetrachloro-2-propene and hexachloropropene by S9 mix via two different metabolic pathways. Mutat Res, **170**: 1-9.

Neudecker T, Stefani A, & Henschler D (1977) *In vitro* mutagenicity of the soil nematicide 1,3-dichloropropene. Experientia (Basel), 33: 1084-1085.

Neudecker T, Lutz D, Eder E, & Henschler D (1980) Structure-activity relationship in halogen and alkyl substituted allyl and allylic compounds: Correlation of alkylating and mutagenic properties. Biochem Pharmacol, 29: 2611-2617.

Neuhauser EF, Loehr RC, & Malecki MR (1985a) Contact and artificial soil tests using earthworms to evaluate the impact of wastes in soil. In: Petros JK Jr, Lacy WJ, & Conway W ed. Hazardous and industrial solid waste: 4th Symposium. Philadelphia, Pennsylvania, American Society for Testing and Materials, pp 192-203 (ASTM Special Technical Publication No. 886).

Neuhauser EF, Loehr RC, Malecki MR, Milligan DL, & Durkin PR (1985b) The toxicity of selected organic chemicals to the earthworm *Eisenia fetida*. J Environ Qual, 14(3): 383-388.

Neuhauser EF, Durkin PR, Malecki MR, & Anatra M (1986) Comparative toxicity of ten organic chemicals to four earthworm species. Comp Biochem Physiol, 83C(1): 197-200.

NIOSH (1985) 1,2-Dichloropropane: Analytical method 1013. In: Eller PM ed. NIOSH Manual of analytical methods. Cincinnati, Ohio, National Institute for Occupational Safety and Health, vol 1, pp 1-4.

Nitschke KD & Lomax LG (1990) *Cis*-1,3-dichloropropene: 2-Week vapor inhalation toxicity study in Fischer 344 rats. Internal report. Midland, Michigan, Dow Chemical Company (Unpublished proprietary report submitted to WHO by Dow Chemical).

Nitschke KD, Johnson KA, Wackerle DL, Phillips JE, & Dittenber DA (1988) Propylene dichloride: 13-Week inhalation toxicity study with rats, mice and rabbits. Internal report. Midland, Michigan, Dow Chemical Company (Unpublished proprietary report submitted to WHO by Dow Chemical).

Nitschke KD, Crissman JW, & Schuetz DJ (1990) *Cis*-1,3-dichloropropene: Acute inhalation study with Fischer 344 rats. Internal report. Midland, Michigan, Dow Chemical Company (Unpublished proprietary report submitted to WHO by Dow Chemical).

Nitschke KD, Lomax LG, & Sanderson TG (1991) *Cis*-1,3-dichloropropene: 13-Week vapor inhalation toxicity study in Fischer 344 rats. Internal report. Midland, Michigan, Dow Chemical Company (Unpublished proprietary report submitted to WHO by Dow Chemical).

NTP (1983) Carcinogenesis bioassay of 1,2-dichloropropane (propylene dichloride) in F344/N rats and $B_6C_3F_1$ mice (gavage study). Research Triangle Park, North Carolina, National Toxicology Program (NTP Technical Report No. 82-092; NIH publication No. 82-2519).

NTP (1985) Toxicology and carcinogenesis studies of Telone II, in F344/N rats and $B_6C_3F_1$ mice (gavage studies). Research Triangle Park, North Carolina, National Toxicology Program (NTP Technical Report No. 269; NIH-publication No. 85-2525).

NTP (1986) Toxicology and carcinogenesis studies of 1,2-dichloropropane (propylene dichloride) in F344/N rats and $B_6C_3F_1$ mice (gavage studies). Research Triangle Park, North Carolina, National Toxicology Program (NTP Technical Report No. 263; NIH Publication No. 86-2519).

O'Connor J (1990a) *Cis*-1,3-dichloropropene: Determination of physico-chemical properties. Eye, United Kingdom, Life Science Research Ltd (Unpublished proprietary report No. 90/SLK005/0461, submitted to WHO by Shell).

O'Connor J (1990b) *Cis*-1,3-dichloropropene: Determination of hydrolysis as a function of pH. Eye, United Kingdom, Life Science Research Ltd (Unpublished proprietary report No. 90/SLK006/0479, submitted to WHO by Shell).

Oldenhuis R, Vink RLJM, Janssen DB, & Witholt B (1989) Degradation of chlorinated aliphatic hydrocarbons by *Methylosinus trichosporium* OB3b expressing soluble methane monooxygenase. Appl Environ Microbiol, **55**(11): 2819-2826.

Onkenhout W, Mulder PPJ, Boogaard PJ, Buys W, & Vermeulen NPE (1986) Identification and quantitative determination of mercapturic acids formed from Z- and E-1,3-dichloropropene by the rat, using gaschromatography with three different detection techniques. Arch Toxicol, **59**: 235-241.

Orrenius S, Thor H, McConkey D, Nicotera P, & Bellomo G (1989) Mechanism of cell toxicity: the thiol/calcium hypothesis. In: Proceedings of the VII International Symposium on Microsomes and Drug Oxidation. London, Taylor & Francis, pp 329-337.

Osterloh J, Letz G, Pond S, & Becker C (1983) An assessment of the potential testicular toxicity of 10 pesticides using the mouse-sperm morphology assay. Mutat Res, **116**: 407-415.

Osterloh JD, Cohen BS, Popendorf W, & Pond SM (1984) Urinary excretion of the N-acetyl cysteine conjugate of *cis*-1,3-dichloropropene by exposed individuals. Arch Environ Health, **39**(4): 271-275.

Osterloh JD, Wang R, Schneider F, & Maddy K (1989) Biological monitoring of dichloropropene: Air concentrations, urinary metabolite, and renal enzyme excretion. Arch Environ Health, **44**(4): 207-213.

O'Sullivan PK, Schweizer AK, & Lu CC (1980) Audit of Industrial Bio-Test Laboratories Study No. 623-06212: Teratogenic study with D-D in albino rats (Regulatory Information Record No. WRC RIR-6). Houston, Texas, Shell Development Company (Unpublished proprietary report submitted to WHO by Shell).

Otson R, Williams DT, & Bothwell PD (1982) Volatile organic compounds in water and thirty Canadian potable water treatment facilities. J Assoc Off Anal Chem, **65**(6): 1370-1374.

Ou L-T (1989) Degradation of Telone II in contaminated and noncontaminated soils. J Environ Sci Health, **B24**(6): 661-574.

Parker CM (1980) Histopathologic evaluation of tissues and organs from beagle dogs in a two-year chronic oral toxicity study fed D-D compound (Regulatory Information Record No. WRC RIR-3). Houston, Texas, Shell Development Company (Unpublished proprietary report submitted to WHO by Shell).

Parker CM, Coate WB, & Voelker RW (1982) Subchronic inhalation toxicity of 1,3-dichloropropene/1,2-dichloropropane (D-D) in mice and rats. J Toxicol Environ Health, **9**: 899-910.

Pearson CR & McConnell G (1975) Chlorinated C_1 and C_2 hydrocarbons in the marine environment. Proc R Soc Lond, **B189**: 305-332.

Peoples SA, Maddy KT, Cusick W, Jackson T, Cooper C, & Frederickson AS (1980) A study of samples of well water collected from selected areas in California to determine the presence of DBCP and certain other pesticide residues. Bull Environ Contam Toxicol, **24**: 611-618.

Perbellini L, Zedda A, Schiavon R, & Franchi GL (1985) [Two cases of disseminated intravascular coagulation syndrome (DIC) caused by exposure to 1,2-dichloropropane (commercial trichloroethylene).] Med Lav, **76**(5): 412-417 (in Italian).

Perocco P, Bolognesi S, & Alberghini W (1983) Toxic activity of seventeen industrial solvents and halogenated compounds on human lymphocytes cultured *in vitro*. Toxicol Lett, **16**: 69-75.

Perry J & Roberts TR (1974) The degradation and leaching of Z and E-3-chloroacrylic acids in soils. Sittingbourne, Shell Research Ltd. (Unpublished proprietary report WKGR 0098.74, submitted to WHO by Shell).

Pochon J, Lajudie J, & Coppier O (1951) Remarques sur les recherches relatives à l'action de certaines substances antiparasitaires sur la microflore du sol. Ann Inst Pasteur, **80**: 517-519.

Ponticelli C, Imbasciati E, Redaelli B, & Salvadeo A (1968) [Acute hepatorenal insufficiency due to trielene.] Lav Um, **20**: 205-212 (in Italian).

Portmann JE & Wilson KW (1971) The toxicity of 140 substances to the Brown shrimp and other marine animals. London, Ministry of Agriculture, Fisheries and Food (Shellfish Information Leaflet No. 22).

Pozzi C, Marai P, Ponti R, Dell'Oro C, Sala C, Zedda S, & Locatelli F (1985) Toxicity in man due to stain removers containing 1,2-dichloropropane. Br J Ind Med, **42**: 770-772.

Price JB & Andrews IJ (1985) The *in vitro* assessment of eye irritancy using enucleated eyes. Food Chem Toxicol, **23**(2): 313-315.

Priston RAJ, Brooks TM, Hodson-Walker G, & Wiggins DE (1983) Genotoxicity studies with 1,2-dichloropropane. Sittingbourne, Shell Research Ltd (Unpublished proprietary report SBGR 83.083, submitted to WHO by Shell).

Rader WE & Love JW (1977a) Impact of commercial Shell products on microorganisms in the soil. Part. I. Effect on modulation on pinto beans and on the nitrogen fixation bacteria (Technical Information Record No. TIR-22-112-77, Part I). Modesto, California, Shell Development Company (Unpublished proprietary report submitted to WHO by Shell).

Rader WE & Love JW (1977b) Impact of commercial Shell pesticides on microorganisms in the soil. Part. II. Effect on decomposition of cellulose in the soil (Technical Information Record No. TIR-22-112-77, Part II). Modesto, California, Shell Development Company (Unpublished proprietary report submitted to WHO by Shell).

Rader WE, Love JW, & Chai EY (1978) Impact of commercial Shell pesticides on microorganisms in the soil. Part III. Effect of compounds on the populations of microorganisms and the O2/CO2 exchange in treated soil (Technical Information Record

No. TIR-22-112-77, Part III). Modesto, California, Shell Development Company (Unpublished proprietary report submitted to WHO by Shell).

Rader WE (1979a) Impact of commercial Shell pesticides on microorganisms in the soil. Part IV. The effect of the compounds on soil nitrification (Technical Information Record No. TIR-22-112-77, Part IV). Modesto, California, Shell Development Company (Unpublished proprietary report submitted to WHO by Shell).

Rader WE (1979b) The effects of Shell pesticides on protein decomposition (Technical Information Record No. TIR-51-108-79). Modesto, California, Shell Development Company (Unpublished proprietary report submitted to WHO by Shell).

Rader WE (1979c) The effect of Shell pesticides on soil phosphatase activity (Technical Information Record No. TIR-51-110-79). Modesto, California, Shell Development Company (Unpublished proprietary report submitted to WHO by Shell).

Rexilius L & Schmidt H (1982) Investigations into the migratory behaviour of 1,3-dichloropropene and methylisothiocyanate in the soil of the nursery areas. Nachrichtenbl Dtsch Pflanzenschutzd, 34(11): 161-165.

Reiff B (1975) Soil fumigant D-D: its toxicity to fish. Sittingbourne, Shell Research Ltd (Unpublished proprietary report TLGR 0035.75, submitted to WHO by Shell).

Reiff B (1978) The acute toxicity of 1,3-dichloropropene to the Golden orfe (*Idus idus melanotus*). Sittingbourne, Shell Research Ltd (Unpublished proprietary report TLGR 0057.78, submitted to WHO by Shell).

Reinert KH, Hunter JV, & Sabatine T (1983) Dynamic heated headspace analysis of volatile organic compounds present in fish tissue samples. J Agric Food Chem, 31: 1057-1060.

Rick DL & McCarty LP (1988) The determination of the odor threshold of Telone(R) II soil fumigant by a new method. Appl Ind Hyg, 3(11): 299-302.

Roberts TR & Stoydin G (1976) The degradation of (Z)-and (E)-1,3-dichloropropenes and 1,2-dichloropropane in soil. Pestic Sci, 7: 325-335.

Rocchi PSJ & Van Sittert NJ (1989) A monitoring study of the exposure to 1,3-dichloropropene during application in France of Shell D-D and Shell D-D 92 nematocide. Internal report. The Hague, Shell Internationale Petroleum Maatschappij B.V. (Unpublished proprietary report submitted to WHO by Shell).

Rosenblum I & Talley W (1979) Evaluation of instrumental behavioural performance of Rhesus monkeys after acute exposure to Telone II. Albany, New York, Institute of Comparative and Human Toxicology (Unpublished proprietary report submitted to WHO by Dow Chemical).

Ross DJ & McNeilly BA (1975) Influence of four nematicides on soil nitrogen mineralisation and nitrogen uptake by white clover in a yellow-grey earth. NZ J Agric Res, 18: 155-162.

Schiffmann D, Eder E, Neudecker T, & Henschler D (1983) Induction of unscheduled DNA synthesis in Hela cells by allylic compounds. Cancer Lett, 20(3): 263-269.

Schuurman P (1989) Physico-chemical properties of *trans*-1,3-dichloropropene. Part II. Rijswijk, The Netherlands, Organization for Applied Scientific Research (Unpublished proprietary report No. PML 1989-C35, submitted to WHO by Shell).

Schweizer AK & Parker CM (1980) Audit of Industrial Bio-test Laboratories Study No. 651-06000: Two-year chronic oral toxicity study with D-D compound in beagle dogs (Regulatory Information Record No. WRC RIR-4). Houston, Texas, Shell Development Company (Unpublished proprietary report submitted to WHO by Shell).

Shell (1976) Determination of residues of 1,2-dichloropropane, 1,3-dichloropropene (Z and E isomers), and 3-chloro-allyl alcohol (Z and E isomers) in crops and soil. Sittingbourne, Shell Research Ltd (Unpublished proprietary report No. WAMS 222-1, submitted to WHO by Shell).

Shell (1978) Residue determination of the E-and Z-isomers of 3-chloroallylalcohol (CAA) in crops and soil. Modesto, California, Shell Development Company (Unpublished proprietary report No. MMS-R-481-1, submitted to WHO by Shell).

Shell (1980) Residue determination of (E) and (Z)-isomers of 3-chloroallylalcohol in agricultural commodities and water. Sittingbourne, Shell Research Ltd (Unpublished proprietary report No. MMS-R-506-1, submitted to WHO by Shell).

Shell (1984) Residue determination of 1,2-dichloropropane and the Z- and E-isomers of 1,3-dichloropropene in agricultural commodities, soil and water. Sittingbourne, Shell Research Ltd (Unpublished proprietary report No. MMS-R-505-3, submitted to WHO by Shell).

Shell (1985) D-D/D-D92. Review of the occurrence and fate of residues in crops and the environment. London, Shell International Chemical Company Ltd, Regulatory Affairs, Crop Protection Division (Unpublished proprietary report submitted to WHO by Shell).

Shell IPM (1990) Review of environmental toxicology D-D92 (1,3-dichloropropene). The Hague, Shell Internationale Petroleum Maatschappij B.V. (Review Series HSE 90.001) (Unpublished proprietary report submitted to WHO by Shell).

Sherren AJ & Woodbridge AP (1987a) "D-D 92" residue and environmental fate studies - Small scale field studies. Internal report. London, Shell Research Ltd (Unpublished proprietary report SBGR 87.170, submitted to WHO by Shell).

Sherren AJ & Woodbridge AP (1987b) "D-D 92" residue and environmental fate studies - Development of air monitoring methods. Internal report. London, Shell Research Ltd (Unpublished proprietary report SBGR 87.141, submitted to WHO by Shell).

Sherren AJ & Woodbridge AP (1987c) "D-D 92" residue and environmental fate studies - Volatilization of "D-D 92" following treatment of soil in an outdoor enclosure. Internal report. London, Shell Research Ltd (Unpublished proprietary report SBGR 87.157, submitted to WHO by Shell).

Sherren AJ (1990) D-D 92 residue and environmental fate studies. Field study - France - Air monitoring. Internal report. London, Shell Research Ltd (Unpublished proprietary report SBGR 89.127, submitted to WHO by Shell).

Shirasu Y, Moriya M, Tezuka H, Teramoto S, Ohta T, & Inoue T (1981) Mutagenicity screening studies on pesticides. In: Environmental mutagens and carcinogens: Proceedings of the Third International Conference on Environmental Mutagens, Tokyo, Mishima and Kyoto, 21-27 September 1981, pp 331-335.

Sittig M (1980) Priority toxic pollutants. Health impacts and allowable limits. Park Ridge, New Jersey, Noyes Data Corporation, pp 192-196.

Smelt JH, Teunissen W, Crum SJH, & Leistra M (1989) Accelerated transformation of 1,3-dichloropropene in loamy soils. Neth J Agric Sci, 37: 173-183.

Smyth HF Jr, Carpenter CP, Weil CS, Pozzani VC, Striegel JA, & Nycum JS (1969) Range-finding toxicity data: List VII. Am Ind Hyg Assoc J, 30(5): 470-476.

Sommer K (1970) [Influence of different pesticides on nitrification and nitrogen transformation in soils.] Landwirtsch Forsch, 25: 22-30 (in German with English summary).

Stevens JL, Ayoubi N, & Robbins JD (1988) The role of mitochondrial matrix enzymes in the metabolism and toxicity of cysteine conjugates. J Biol Chem, 263: 3395-3401.

Stolzenberg SJ & Hine CH (1980) Mutagenicity of 2- and 3-carbon halogenated compounds in the *Salmonella*/mammalian microsome test. Environ Mutagen, 2(1): 59-66.

Stott WT & Kastl PE (1985) Inhalation pharmacokinetics of technical grade 1,3-dichloropropene in rats. Internal report. Midland, Michigan, Dow Chemical Company (Unpublished proprietary report submitted to WHO by Dow Chemical).

Stott WT & Kastl PE (1986) Inhalation pharmacokinetics of technical grade 1,3-dichloropropene in rats. Toxicol Appl Pharmacol, 85(3): 332-341.

Stott WT, Young JT, Calhoun LL, & Battjes JE (1984) Telone II, soil fumigant: 13-week inhalation study in rats and mice. Internal report. Midland, Michigan, Dow Chemical Company (Unpublished proprietary report submitted to WHO by Dow Chemical).

Stott WT, Johnson KA, Calhoun LL, Weiss SK, & Franson LE (1987) Telone II soil fumigant: 2-year inhalation chronic toxicity-oncogenicity study in mice (Study No. M-003993-009). Midland, Michigan Dow Chemical Company (Unpublished proprietary report submitted to WHO by Dow Chemical).

Stott WT, Young JT, Calhoun LL, & Battjes JE (1988) Subchronic toxicity of inhaled technical grade 1,3-dichloropropene in rats and mice. Fundam Appl Toxicol, 11: 207-220.

Stott WT, Waechter JM, & Quast JT (1990) Letter to the editor. Arch Environ Health, 45: 250-253.

Straley JP, Christiansen JA, & Kopecky AL (1982) Improved biological degradation chlorinated hydrocarbons using mutant bacteria. Proc Int Water Conf Eng Soc West, 43: 523-531.

Streeter CM, Battjes JE, & Lomax LG (1987) Telone II soil fumigant. An acute vapor inhalation study in Fischer 344 rats. Internal report. Midland, Michigan, Dow Chemical Company (Unpublished proprietary report submitted to WHO by Dow Chemical).

Sullivan DA, Jones AD, & Williams JG (1985) Results of the US Environmental Protection Agency's air toxics analysis in Philadelphia (Prepared for presentation at the 78th Annual Meeting of the Air Pollution Control Association, Detroit, Michigan, 16-21 June 1985). Washington, DC, US Environmental Protection Agency, pp 1-15 (Report 85-17.5).

Tabak HH, Quave SA, Mashni CI, & Barth EF (1981) Biodegradability studies with organic priority pollutant compounds. J Water Pollut Control Fed, **53**: 1503.

Talcott RE & King J (1984) Mutagenic impurities in 1,3-dichloropropene preparations. J Natl Cancer Inst, 72(5): 1113-1116.

Telliard WA (1990) Broad-range methods for determination of pollutants in wastewater. J Chromatogr Sci, **28**: 453-459.

Thomason IJ & McKenry MV (1974) Part I. Movement and fate as affected by various conditions in several soils. Hilgardia, **42**: 392-420.

Thorel JM, Bercoff E, Massari Ph, Droy JM, Chassagne Ph, Proust B, Hemet J, & Bourreille J (1986) Toxicité du 1,2-dichloropropane: à propos d'un cas avec hypertension portale. J Toxicol Clin Exp, 6(4): 247-252.

Thornton GD (1951) Some effects of D-D, EDB and chloropicrin on microbiological action in several Florida soils. Proc Soil Sci Soc Florida, **1951**(11): 68-71.

Til HP, Spanjers MTh, Feron VJ, & Renzel PJG (1973) Sub-chronic (90-day) toxicity study with Telone in albino rats (Final report). Zeist, The Netherlands, Central Institute for Nutrition and Food Research (Unpublished proprietary report No. R-4002, submitted to WHO by Dow Chemical).

Timchalk C, Bartels MJ, Dryzga MD, & Smith FA (1989) Propylene dichloride: Pharmacokinetics and metabolism in Fischer 344 rats following oral and inhalation exposure. Internal report. Midland, Michigan, Dow Chemical Company (Unpublished proprietary report submitted to WHO by Dow Chemical).

Torkelson TR & Oyen F (1977) The toxicity of 1,3-dichloropropene as determined by repeated exposure of laboratory animals. Am Ind Hyg Assoc J, **38**: 217-223.

Toyoshima S, Sato R, & Sato S (1978a) The acute toxicity test of Telone II in mice (Unpublished proprietary report submitted to WHO by Dow Chemical).

Toyoshima S, Sato R, & Sato S (1978b) The acute toxicity test of Telone II in rats. (Unpublished proprietary report submitted to WHO by Dow Chemical).

Trevisan A, Rizzi E, Bungaro A, Pozzobon L, Gioffre F, Scapinello A, Valeri A, & Chiesura P (1988) Proximal tubule brush border angiotensin converting enzyme behaviour and nephrotoxicity due to 1,2-dichloropropane. The target organ and the toxic process. Arch Toxicol, **12**(Suppl): 190-192.

Trevisan A, Rizzi E, Scapinello A, Gioffre F, & Chiesura P (1989) Liver toxicity due to 1,2-dichloropropane in the rat. Arch Toxicol, **63**: 445-449.

Trevisan A, Troso O, & Maso S (1991) Recovery of biochemical changes induced by 1,2-dichloropropane in rat liver and kidney. Hum Exp Toxicol, **10**: 241-244.

Tu CM (1972) Effects of four nematocides on activities of microorganisms in soil. Appl Microbiol, 23(2): 398-401.

Tu CM (1973) Effects of Mocap. N-Serve, Telone, and Vorlex at two temperatures on populations and activities of microorganisms in soil. Can J Plant Sci, 53: 401-405.

Tu CM (1978) Effect of pesticides on acetylene reduction and microorganisms in a sandy loam. Soil Biol Biochem, 10: 451-456.

Tu CM (1979) Influence of pesticides on acetylene reduction and growth of microorganisms in an organic soil. J Environ Sci Health, B14(6): 617-624.

Tu CM (1981a) Effects of pesticides on activities of enzymes and microorganisms in a clay soil. J Environ Sci Health, B16(2): 179-191.

Tu CM (1981b) Effects of some pesticides on enzyme activities in an organic soil. Bull Environ Contam Toxicol, 27: 109-114.

Tu CM (1988) Effects of selected pesticides on activities of invertase, amylase and microbial respiration in sandy soil. Chemosphere, 17(1): 159-163.

Tuazon EC, Atkinson R, Winer AM, & Pitts JN Jr (1984) A study of the atmospheric reactions of 1,3-dichloropropene and other selected organochlorine compounds. Arch Environ Contam Toxicol, 13: 691-700.

US EPA (1980) Ambient water quality criteria for dichloropropane and dichloropropene. Washington, DC, US Environmental Protection Agency, Office of Water Regulations and Standards Criteria (Report No. 440/5-80-043, PB 81-117541).

US EPA (1985) Health and environmental effects profile for 1,3-dichloropropene. US Cincinnati, Ohio, Environmental Protection Agency, Environmental Criteria and Assessment Office (EPA/600/X-85-399).

US EPA (1990) Inhalation reference concentration for 1,3-dichloropropene (542-75-6). Fairfax, Virginia, Clement International Corporation (Prepared for the US Environmental Protection Agency, Washington).

US EPA (1991) 1,3-Dichloropropene. CAS No. 542-75-6. Washington, DC, US Environmental Protection Agency (Unpublished report).

Valencia R, Mason JM, Woodruff RC, & Zimmering S (1985) Chemical mutagenesis testing in Drosophila. III. Results of 48 coded compounds tested for the National Toxicology Program. Environ Mutagen, 7: 325-348.

Van Beek CGEM, Janssen HMJ, & Puijker LM (1988) [Pesticides in groundwater.] H_2O, 21(4): 80-85 (in Dutch).

Van Den Berg F & Leistra M (1989) Behaviour of the fumigant 1,3-dichloropropene in soil and its emission into the air. Internal report. Wageningen, The Netherlands, The Winand Staring Centre for Integrated Land, Soil and Water Research.

Van Den Brande J & Heungens A (1969) Influence of repeated applications of nematicides on the soil fauna in *Begonia* culture. Neth J Plant Pathol, 75: 40-44.

Van Der Pas LJT & Leistra M (1987) Movement and transformation of 1,3-dichloropropene in the soil of flower-bulb fields. Arch Environ Contam Toxicol, 16: 417-422.

Van Dijk H (1974) Degradation of 1,3-dichloropropenes in the soil. Agro-ecosystems, 1: 193-204.

Van Dijk H (1980) Dissipation rates in soil of 1,2-dichloropropane and 1,3- and 2,3-dichloropropenes. Pestic Sci, 11: 625-632.

Van Duuren BL, Goldschmidt BM, Loevengart G, Smith AC, Melchionne S, Seidman I, & Roth D (1979) Carcinogenicity of halogenated olefinic and aliphatic hydrocarbons in mice. J Natl Cancer Inst, 63(6): 1433-1439.

Van Duuren BL, Kline SA, Melchionne S, & Seidman J (1983) Chemical structure and carcinogenicity relationships of some chloroalkene oxides and their parent olefins. Cancer Res, 43: 159-162.

Van Hooidonk C (1989) Physico-chemical properties of *trans*-1,3-dichloropropene. Rijswijk, The Netherlands, Organization for Applied Scientific Research (Unpublished proprietary report PML 1989-C118, submitted to WHO by Shell).

Van Joost Th & De Jong G (1988) Sensitization to DD soil fumigant during manufacture. Contact Dermatitis, 18(5): 307-308.

Van Sittert NJ (1978) D-D monitoring studies on field workers in France. The Hague, Shell Internationale Petroleum Maatschappij B.V. (Unpublished proprietary report TOX 78-001, submitted to WHO by Shell).

Van Sittert NJ (1984) Biomonitoring of chemicals and their metabolites. In: Berlin A, Draper M, Hemminki K, & Vainio H ed. Monitoring human exposure to carcinogenic and mutagenic agents. Lyon, International Agency for Research on Cancer, pp 153-172 (IARC Scientific Publications No. 59).

Van Sittert NJ (1989) Individual exposure monitoring from plasma or urinary metabolite determination. Arch Toxicol 13(Suppl): 91-100.

Van Sittert NJ, Van der Harst J, & Verhoeven PF (1977) D-D monitoring studies on field workers in Holland. The Hague, Shell Internationale Petroleum Maatschappij B.V. (Unpublished proprietary report TOX 77-001, submitted to WHO by Shell).

Van Welie RTH, Van Duyn P, & Vermeulen NPE (1989) Determination of two mercapturic acid metabolites of 1,3-dichloropropene in human urine with gas chromatography and sulphur-selective detection. J Chromatogr, 496: 463-471.

Van Welie RTH, Van Duyn P, Brouwer DH, Van Hemmen JJ, Brouwer EJ, & Vermeulen NPE (1991) Inhalation exposure to 1,3-dichloropropene in the Dutch flower-bulb culture. Part.II. Biological monitoring by measurement of urinary excretion of two mercapturic acid metabolites. Arch Environ Contam Toxicol, 20: 6-12.

Varanka I (1979) Effect of some pesticides on the rhythmic adductor muscle activity of fresh-water mussel larvae. Symp Biol Hung, 19: 177-196.

Venable JR, McClimans CD, Flake RE, & Dimick DB (1980) A fertility study of male employees engaged in the manufacture of glycerine. J Occup Med, 22(2): 87-91.

Vithayathil AJ, McClure C, & Myers JW (1983) *Salmonella*/microsome multiple indicator mutagenicity test. Mutat Res, 121:(1) 33-37.

Von Der Hude W, Scheutwinkel M, Gramlich U, Fiszler B, & Basler A (1987) Genotoxicity of three-carbon compounds evaluated in the SCE test *in vitro*. Environ Mutagen, 9: 401-410.

Von Der Hude W, Behm C, Gurtler R, & Basler A (1988) Evaluation of the SOS chromotest. Mutat Res, 203: 81-94.

Waechter JM Jr & Kastl PE (1988) 1,3-Dichloropropene: Pharmacokinetics and metabolism in Fischer 344 rats following repeated oral administration. Internal report. Midland, Michigan, Dow Chemical Company, (Unpublished proprietary report submitted to WHO by Dow Chemical).

Wallbridge CT, Fiandt JT, Phipps GL, & Holcombe GW (1983) Acute toxicity of ten chlorinated aliphatic hydrocarbons to the fathead minnow (*Pimephales promelas*). Arch Environ Contam Toxicol, 12: 661-666.

Walker AIT (1968a) The toxicity of D-D soil fumigant (1,2-dichloropropane: 1,3-dichloropropene). 13-week oral toxicity experiment in rats. Sittingbourne, Shell Research Ltd (Unpublished proprietary report TLGR 0018.68, submitted to WHO by Shell).

Walker AIT (1968b) The toxicity of D-D soil fumigant (1,2-dichloropropane: 1,3-dichloropropene). 13-week oral toxicity experiment in dogs. Sittingbourne, Shell Research Ltd (Unpublished proprietary report TLGR 0019.68, submitted to WHO by Shell).

Wallace BG (1974) Development of methods for the determination of residues of free and bound 3-chloroallylalcohol in soil and crops. London, Shell Research Ltd (Unpublished proprietary report WKGR 0067.74, submitted to WHO by Shell).

Wallace BG (1976a) Residues of the major components of D-D and primary metabolites in soil from Germany. London, Shell Research Ltd (Unpublished proprietary report WKGR 0051.76, submitted to WHO by Shell).

Wallace BG (1976b) Residues of the major components of D-D and primary metabolites in soil and crops from Holland. London, Shell Research Ltd (Unpublished proprietary report WKGR 0052.76, submitted to WHO by Shell).

Wallace BG (1979) Residues of D-D and 1,3-D in soil from the UK. London, Shell Research Ltd (Unpublished proprietary report BLGR 79.093, submitted to WHO by Shell).

Watson WP, Lang KL, Brooks TM, Huckle KR, & Wright AS (1986a) Genotoxicity studies with (Z)-1,3-dichloropropene: Mutagenic contaminants. Sittingbourne, Shell Research Ltd (Unpublished proprietary report SBGR 85.246, submitted to WHO by Shell).

Watson WP, Lang KL, Brooks TM, & Wright AS (1986b) Genotoxicity studies with (Z)-1,3-dichloropropene: Bioactivation by mammalian mono-oxygenases and the protective role of glutathione. Sittingbourne, Shell Research Ltd (Unpublished proprietary report SBGR 86.056, submitted to WHO by Shell).

Watson WP, Brooks TM, Huckle KR, Hutson DH, Lang KL, Smith RJ, & Wright AS (1987) Microbial mutagenicity studies with (Z)-1,3-dichloropropene. Chem-Biol Interact, 61: 17-30.

Wensley RN (1953) Microbiological studies of the action of some selected soil fumigants. Can J Bot, **31**: 277-308.

WHO (in preparation) Guidelines for drinking-water quality, 2nd ed. Geneva, World Health Organization.

Williams IH (1968) Recovery of *cis*- and *trans*-dichloropropene residues from 2 types of soil and their detection and determination by electron capture gas chromatography. J Econ Entomol, **61**(5): 1432-1435.

Woodruff RC, Mason JM, Valencia R, & Zimmering S (1985) Chemical mutagenesis testing in *Drosophila*. V. Results of 53 coded compounds tested for the National Toxicology Program. Environ Mutagen, **7**: 677-702.

Worthing CR & Hance RJ (1991) The pesticide manual: A world compendium, 9th ed. Croydon, The British Crop Protection Council, pp 254-255.

Wright AS & Creedy CL (1982) The protective action of glutathione on the microbial mutagenicity of (Z)-1,3-dichloropropene. Sittingbourne, Shell Research Ltd (Unpublished proprietary report SBGR 81.317, submitted to WHO by Shell).

Yakel HO & Kociba RJ (1977) Acute inhalation toxicity of M-3993 (Telone II) in rats. Internal report. Midland, Michigan, Dow Chemical Company (Unpublished proprietary report submitted to WHO by Dow Chemical).

Yang RSH (1986) 1,3-Dichloropropene. Residue Rev, **97**: 19-35.

Yang RSH, Huff JE, Boorman GA, Haseman JK, Kornreich M, & Stookey JL (1986) Chronic toxicology and carcinogenesis studies of Telone II by gavage in Fischer 344 rats and $B_6C_3F_1$ mice. J Toxicol Environ Health, **18**: 377-392.

Yano BL, Calhoun LL, Stott W, Johnson KA, & Schuetz DJ (1985) Telone II soil fumigant: 2 year inhalation chronic toxicity-oncogenicity study in mice. Interim report: 6- and 12-month exposures. Internal report. Midland, Michigan, Dow Chemical Company (Unpublished proprietary report submitted to WHO by Dow Chemical).

Yon DA, Morrison GA, & McGibbon, A.S. (1991) The dissipation of 1,3-dichloropropene in ditch bottom sediment and associated aerobic ditch water. Pestic Sci, **32**: 147-159.

RESUME ET EVALUATION, CONCLUSIONS, ET RECOMMANDATIONS
1,3-DICHLOROPROPENE

1. Résumé et évaluation

1.1 Usage, destinée et concentrations dans l'environnement

Le "1,3-dichloropropène" a été introduit en agriculture en 1956, mélangé à des 1,3-dichloropropènes, du 1,2-dichloropropane et d'autres hydrocarbures halogénés. On l'utilise depuis largement comme fumigant du sol avant plantation pour lutter contre les nématodes qui parasitent les légumes, les pommes de terre et le tabac. L'application s'effectue essentiellement par injection dans le sol. La formulation du commerce consiste en un mélange d'isomères *cis* et *trans* (en proportions approximativement égales), et se présente sous la forme d'un liquide incolore à ambré dont l'odeur pénétrante et irritante rappelle celle du chloroforme. Sa tension de vapeur est de 3.7 kPa à 20 °C. Le produit technique a une pureté de 92% et peut contenir certaines impuretés, comme le 1,2-dichloropropane. Le coefficient de partage octanol/eau (log K_{ow}) est égal à 1,98.

Dans l'air, la décomposition du 1,3-dichloropropène s'effectue principalement par réaction avec des radicaux libres et l'ozone. Dans le cas de la réaction avec les radicaux libres, la demi-vie des isomères *cis*- et *trans*- est respectivement égale à 12 et 7 heures et dans le cas de la réaction avec l'ozone, de 52 et 12 jours. Il semble que la phototransformation directe soit négligeable mais elle pourrait être favorisée par la présence de particules en suspension dans l'atmosphère.

Dans l'eau, il est probable que le 1,3-dichloropropène disparaît rapidement du fait de sa solubilité relativement faible et de sa forte volatilité; on a fait état d'une demi-vie de moins de 5 heures.

La distribution du 1,3-dichloropropène dans les différents compartiments du sol dépend de la tension de vapeur, du coefficient de diffusion, de la température et de la teneur en eau. La persistance du 1,3-dichloropropène dans le sol dépend de sa volatilisation, des transformations chimiques, photo-chimiques ou biologiques qu'il subit et de sa fixation par les êtres vivants. La volatilisation et la diffusion en phase gazeuse sont les mécanismes les plus importants de sa dispersion et de la dilution dans le milieu.

Dans l'environnement, la transformation du 1,3-dichloropropène commence par une hydrolyse en alcool 3-chloro-allylique puis, sous l'action des microorganismes, en 3-chloro-acroléine et en acide 3-chloro-acrylique. Une étude de laboratoire a montré que le temps de demi-hydrolyse des isomères *cis*- et *trans*- du 1,3-dichloropropène à 15 °C et à 29 °C était respectivement égal, pour l'isomère *cis*, à 11 et 2 jours et pour l'isomère *trans*, à 13 et 2 jours. Dans le sol, à un pH de 7, on a observé un temps de demi-hydrolyse à 25 °C de 4,6 jours pour les deux isomères. Du fait que le composé disparaît relativement vite du sol, il est peu probable que des résidus s'y accumulent après application du fumigant à la dose et selon la périodicité recommandées.

Le 1,3-dichloropropène est potentiellement mobile dans le sol, en particulier dans les sols sableux à texture lâche dont la teneur en eau est faible. Son cheminement en profondeur est favorisé par les cultures profondes dans des sols de faible porosité. On a décelé du 1,3-dichloropropène dans les nappes souterraines peu profondes (jusqu'à 2 m en-dessous de la surface) mais non dans les eaux profondes, c'est-à-dire celles qui ont le plus de chances d'être utilisées pour la consommation humaine.

Le 1,3-dichloropropène peut-être fixé par les plantes cultivées. Toutefois, il est peu probable qu'il donne lieu à des résidus importants dans les cultures vivrières car celles-ci sont en principe plantées lorsque la majeure partie du fumigant s'est dissipée.

La bioaccumulation du 1,3-dichloropropène est peu probable car il possède une solubilité dans l'eau relativement forte (> 1 g/kg), un coefficient de partage octanol/eau faible (log K_{ow}) et il est rapidement éliminé chez les mammifères et autres organismes.

1.2 Cinétique et métabolisme

Après administration par voie orale à des rongeurs, le 1,3-dichloropropène est rapidement éliminé. La principale voie d'élimination est la voie urinaire, avec 81% de l'isomère *cis* et 56% de l'isomère de *trans* excrétés dans les 24 heures suivant l'administration. La demi-vie d'élimination dans l'urine est de 5 à 6 heures. L'élimination dans les matières fécales est minime. Le 1,3-dichloropropène est éliminé à hauteur de 4% (isomère *cis*) et de 24% (isomère *trans*) dans le dioxyde de carbone expiré. Après l'administration, les concentrations tissulaires sont faibles; les concentrations résiduelles les plus élevées se retrouvent dans la paroi gastrique, puis, à des valeurs plus faibles, dans les reins, le foie et la vessie.

On ne retrouve pas de 1,3-dichloropropène non modifié dans les urines. Les isomères *cis* et *trans* tiennent lieu de substrats à la glutathion-*S*-alkyltransférase hépatique qui les transforme en acides mercapturiques, excrétés ensuite dans les urines. Le principal métabolite urinaire chez le rat et la souris est la *N*-acétyl-*S*-(3-chloroprop-2-ényl)L-cystéine; ce composé peut être utilisé pour la surveillance biologique chez l'homme. On a observé une deuxième voie métabolique d'importance secondaire dans le cas de l'isomère *cis*; il s'agit d'une mono-oxygénation en *cis*-1,3-dichloropropène oxyde, composé qui peut ensuite être conjugué avec le glutathion. La forte proportion d'isomère *trans* présente dans l'air expiré résulte d'une autre voie métabolique conduisant à la conjugaison, voie qui est plus spécifique de l'isomère *trans* que de l'isomère *cis*.

Exposés par voie respiratoire à du 1,3-dichloropropène, des rats n'ont pas présenté une augmentation du taux sanguin proportionnelle à la dose. A la dose de 408,6 mg/m^3 (90 ppm), la fréquence respiratoire et le volume expiratoire-minute étaient réduits et l'on notait une saturation du métabolisme à 1362 mg/m^3 (300 ppm). Les isomères *cis* et *trans* ont été rapidement éliminés du courant sanguin, avec une demi-vie d'élimination de 3 à 6 minutes pour des concentrations inférieures à 1362 mg/m^3, mais beaucoup plus longue (33 à 43 minutes) à plus forte concentration.

1.3 Effets sur les êtres vivant dans leur milieu naturel

Les valeurs de la CE_{50} relatives à la croissance (à 96 h) chez une algue d'eau douce, *Selenastrum capricornutum*, et chez une diatomée estuarielle, *Skeletoneria costatum*, sont respectivement égales à 4,95 mg/litre et 1 mg/litre. Pour les poissons, la toxicité aiguë du 1,3-dichloropropène (CL_{50} à 96 h), est de l'ordre de 1 à 7,9 mg/litre. Un test effectué sur les stades embryo-larvaires d'un vairon, *Pimephales promelas*, ont donné une dose maximale sans effet observable de 0,24 mg/litre. Ces données, jointes au fait que le 1,3-dichloropropène ne persiste vraisemblablement pas dans l'eau, indiquent que le danger pour les poissons réside dans les effets toxiques aigus de ce composé, mais qu'il y a peu de risques d'effets supplémentaires résultant d'une exposition à long terme.

Aux doses de 30 à 60 mg/kg, le 1,3-dichloropropène peut réduire l'abondance des champignons et l'activité des enzymes microbiennes, mais cet effet n'est généralement pas de longue durée (< 7 jours) et ne se produit pas dans tous les types de sol. Certaines études ont fait ressortir un accroissement sensible du nombre de microorganismes après application du fumigant.

Le 1,3-dichloropropène est phytotoxique mais en revanche, il est peu toxique pour les abeilles. On a constaté, en épandant du 1,3-dichloropropène par poudrage, que la DL_{50} à 48 h était de 6,6 µg/abeille. Les oiseaux sont relativement insensibles au 1,3-dichloropropène. La CL_{50} (8 jours) est inférieure à 10 g/kg de nourriture pour le col-vert et les cailles du genre *Colinis*.

1.4 Effets sur les animaux d'expérience et les systèmes d'épreuve in vitro

La toxicité aiguë par voie orale du 1,3-dichloropropène est modérée à forte chez les animaux d'expérience. En ce qui concerne le rat, on a fait état, pour la DL_{50}, de valeurs se situant entre 127 et 713 mg/kg de poids corporel. Par voie orale, ces valeurs étaient respectivement de 85 et 94 mg/kg de poids corporel pour les isomères *cis* et *trans*.

En cas d'exposition cutanée, le composé est modérément toxique. Chez le rat et le lapin, on a obtenu pour la DL_{50} des valeurs respectivement égales à 423 et 504 mg/kg de poids corporel. Ces valeurs étaient respectivement de 1090 mg pour l'isomère *cis* et de 1575 mg/kg de poids corporel pour l'isomère *trans*.

Chez des rats exposés pendant 4 h par la voie respiratoire à du 1,3-dichloropropène, on a obtenu une CL_{50} de 3310 mg/m^3 (729 ppm); les valeurs allaient de 3042 mg/m^3 à 3514 mg/m^3 pour l'isomère *cis* et de 4880 mg/m^3 à 5403 mg/m^3 pour l'isomère *trans*.

En cas d'intoxication aiguë, on observe une atteinte nerveuse centrale et une atteinte respiratoire.

Des réactions graves ont été observées chez le lapin lors d'épreuves d'irritation cutanée et oculaire mais les animaux ont récupéré en l'espace de 14 à 21 jours. Les épreuves de sensibilisation cutanée chez le cobaye se sont révélées positives.

Plusieurs études de toxicité respiratoire à court terme ont été effectuées sur des souris, des rats, des cobayes, des lapins et des chiens. Chez la souris, c'est les muqueuses nasales et la vessie qui étaient les organes cibles. On a observé une dégénérescence de l'épithélium olfactif et une hyperplasie de l'épithélium respiratoire. Au niveau de la vessie, on a observé une hyperplasie modérée de l'épithélium de transition. On a pu fixer à 136 mg/kg, soit 30 ppm, la dose sans effet observable chez la souris.

Chez le rat, on a observé également une hyperplasie ainsi que des modifications dégénératives analogues au niveau de l'épithélium olfactif. Une étude bien conçue a permis d'obtenir une valeur de 4,35 mg/m^3 pour la dose sans effet observable; dans le cas précis de l'isomère *cis*, cette dose était égale à 136 mg/m^3.

Une étude de 90 jours consistant à administrer le composé par voie orale à des rats a permis de fixer à 3 mg/kg de poids corporel la dose sans effet observable. Le seul effet observé à la dose immédiatement supérieure (10 mg/kg de poids corporel) consistait en une augmentation du poids relatif des reins chez les mâles.

Une étude de reproduction portant sur deux générations et deux portées de rats, à des doses allant jusqu'à 408,6 mg/m^3 (90 ppm), n'a pas fait ressortir d'effets indésirables sur les paramètres examinés. Toutefois, la dose la plus forte (408,6 mg/m^3) était toxique pour les mères, comme l'ont montré les deux anomalies observées: réduction de la croissance et modification histopathologique au niveau de la muqueuse nasale. Les résultats de cette étude ont permis de fixer à 136,2 mg/m^3 (30 ppm) la dose maximale sans effet toxique observable chez les mères.

Des études de tératogénicité au cours desquelles du 1,3-dichloropropène a été administré à des rats et à des lapins par la voie respiratoire, n'ont pas permis de relever d'indices de tératogénicité jusqu'à la dose de 1362 mg/m^3, mais on a observé une embryotoxicité chez le rat (réduction de la taille des portées et augmentation du taux de résorption). Le composé s'est révélé toxique pour les mères, tant chez les rattes que chez les lapines, aux doses supérieures ou égales à 544,8 mg/m^3 (120 ppm).

Dans la plupart des études, les isomères *cis* et *trans* du 1,3-dichloropropène, ainsi que les mélanges, se sont révélés mutagènes chez les bactéries, sans ou avec activation métabolique. A l'état pur, le 1,3-dichloropropène et le *cis*-1,3-dichloropropène étaient négatifs à cet égard chez les bactéries. On a montré que le glutathion bloquait l'activité mutagène du 1,3-dichloropropène chez les bactéries. Lors d'une épreuve de mutation génique sur des cellules V79 de hamster chinois ainsi que dans une épreuve HGPRT sur des cellules ovariennes du même animal, le *cis*-1,3-dichloropropène a donné des résultats négatifs.

Le *cis*- et le *trans*-1,3-dichloropropène provoquent une synthèse non programmée de l'ADN dans les cellules HeLa S$_3$. Dans des hépatocytes de rat, le 1,3-dichloropropène n'a pas entraîné de réparation importante de l'ADN. L'épreuve rec sur des microsomes de la souche H17 de *Bacillus subtilis* a donné un résultat positif avec le 1,3-dichloropropène en présence d'activation métabolique.

Dans des cellules ovariennes de hamster chinois, le *cis*- et le *trans*-1,3-dichloropropène ont entraîné des lésions chromosomiques en présence d'activation métabolique; toutefois dans une autre étude, le 1,3-dichloropropène a produit les mêmes effets sans activation métabolique. Le *cis*-1,3-dichloropropène n'a pas provoqué de lésions chromosomiques dans des cellules de foie de rat, mais il a entraîné des échanges entre chromatides soeurs dans des cellules ovariennes de hamster chinois, en présence ou en l'absence d'activation métabolique, ainsi que dans des cellules V79 du même animal, cette fois sans activation métabolique.

Une épreuve de recherche des micronoyaux dans la moelle osseuse de souris a donné des résultats négatifs avec le 1,3-dichloropropène. Les résultats ont été également négatifs dans le cas d'une épreuve de mutation létale récessive liée au sexe sur *Drosophila melanogaster*.

Des études de cancérogénicité ont été effectuées sur des souris et des rats. On leur a administré par gavage pendant deux ans du 1,3-dichloropropène technique contenant 1% d'épichlorhydrine. Chez les souris, on a noté un accroissement sensible des hyperplasies épithéliales ainsi que des carcinomes de type transitionnel au niveau de la vessie, un accroissement des tumeurs pulmonaires, une légère augmentation des tumeurs hépatiques et, au niveau de la portion cardiaque de l'estomac, une augmentation de l'hyperplasie épithéliale ainsi que des papillomes ou des carcinomes spino-cellulaires. Chez le rat, on a observé une augmentation de l'incidence des nodules néoplasiques au niveau du foie ainsi que des papillomes ou des carcinomes spino-cellulaires dans la portion cardiaque de l'estomac.

Une étude par inhalation de deux ans a permis d'étudier la cancérogénicité du 1,3-dichloropropène (sans épichlorhydrine) sur des rats et des souris. Chez les souris, on a observé une incidence accrue des hyperplasies, au niveau de la vessie, de la portion cardiaque de l'estomac et des muqueuses nasales. Il y avait également augmentation dans l'incidence des tumeurs pulmonaires bénignes. Un certain nombre de modifications d'origine toxique ont été constatées dans la muqueuse olfactive nasale chez le rat, mais sans accroissement de l'incidence tumorale.

On a montré que l'épichlorhydrine provoquait des tumeurs de la partie proximale de l'estomac lors d'une étude où cette substance était administrée par gavage ainsi que des tumeurs des fosses nasales lors d'une étude par inhalation sur des rats; les résultats de l'étude au cours de laquelle du 1,3-dichloropropène a été administré par voie orale à des souris ne permettent pas d'exclure un effet cancérogène sur la vessie.

Mode d'action

Etant donné que la principale voie métabolique d'élimination du 1,3-dichloropropène consiste dans une conjugaison avec le glutathion, on peut penser que toute situation affectant la concentration en glutathion tissulaire (groupements sulfhydriles non protéiques) est susceptible de modifier les effets du composé. Le 1,3-dichloropropène lui-même provoque une déplétion en glutathion dans les divers tissus, en particulier ceux qui constituent la porte d'entrée dans l'organisme, c'est-à-dire essentiellement la portion cardiaque de l'estomac et le foie dans le cas où l'administration se fait par gavage et les tissus des fosses nasales dans le cas des études par inhalation. On a observé chez la souris une diminution du glutathion, au niveau de l'épithélium nasal aux doses supérieurs 22,7 mg/m^3 (5 ppm) et au niveau de la portion cardiaque de l'estomac aux doses supérieurs à 113,5 mg/m^3 (25 ppm).

La toxicité du 1,3-dichloropropène pour les animaux d'expérience se manifeste lorsque l'exposition entraîne une déplétion en glutathion et une réduction préalable de la teneur en glutathion tissulaire exacerbe cet effet toxique. L'inhalation pendant une longue période de concentrations supérieures à 90,8 mg/m^3 (20 ppm) entraîne une dégénérescence et une hyperplasie de l'épithélium nasal et stomacal chez la souris; chez le rat et dans les mêmes conditions, la dose de 272,4 mg/m^3 (60 ppm) a également provoqué une dégénérescence du tissu des fosses nasales.

Le rôle protecteur du glutathion a également été mis en lumière par des études chez la souris qui ont montré que lorsque la teneur en groupements sulfhydriles non protéiques diminuait, il y avait augmentation du taux de liaison covalente du dichloropropène radiomarqué (au carbone 14) aux cellules de la portion cardiaque de l'estomac. De même, on a observé, dans des systèmes d'épreuves *in vitro*, que la présence de glutathion réduisait sensiblement la génotoxicité du 1,3-dichloropropène et d'un des ses métabolites mineurs d'oxydation (cytochrome P-450), à savoir le 1,3-dichloropropène-oxyde.

1.5 Effets sur l'homme

Il est improbable qu'il y ait exposition de la population générale par l'intermédiaire de l'air, de l'eau ou des aliments.

On a montré que l'exposition professionnelle se situe en général en-dessous de 4,54 mg/m^3 (1 ppm), mais on a également fait état de concentrations plus élevées (jusqu'à 18,3 mg/m^3 lors d'opérations de remplissage ou de changement de buses). L'exposition professionnelle se produit vraisemblablement par la voie respiratoire ou par la voie cutanée. Très peu de temps après l'exposition, il y a irritation des yeux et des muqueuses des voies respiratoires supérieures. On a observé de graves symptômes d'intoxication après inhalation d'air contenant des concentrations supérieures à 6810 mg/m^3 (> 1500 ppm); à plus faible concentration, il y avait dépression du système nerveux central et irritation des voies respiratoires. L'exposition de la peau entraîne également de graves irritations à ce niveau.

Chez un groupe de personnes chargées d'épandre du 1,3-dichloropropène, on a observé en fin de saison un certain nombre d'anomalies de la fonction hépatique et rénale. Toutefois, l'existence d'une relation de cause à effet reste controversée.

Il y a eu des cas d'intoxication qui ont entraîné l'hospitalisation des intéressés avec des symptômes d'irritation des muqueuses, une sensation de gêne thoracique, des maux de tête, des nausées, des vomissements, des vertiges et parfois une perte de conscience et une diminution de la libido. En outre, trois cas d'affections hématologiques malignes ont été attribués à une surexposition accidentelle antérieure au 1,3-dichloropropène, mais là encore, l'existence d'une relation de cause à effet reste incertaine.

En comparant à un groupe témoin la fécondité d'employés travaillant à la production d'hydrocarbures chlorés à trois atomes de carbone, on n'a pas mis en évidence d'association entre l'exposition et une réduction éventuelle de la fécondité.

2. Conclusions

Population générale: Du fait que l'exposition au 1,3-dichloropropène est faible voire inexistante, le risque pour la population générale est négligeable.

Exposition professionnelle: Lors d'opérations de remplissage et lors des épandages, il peut y avoir exposition des opérateurs à des concentrations dépassant la limite maximale autorisée, si des mesures de sécurité appropriées ne sont pas prises.

Environnement: Dans la mesure où le 1,3-dichloropropène est utilisé à la dose recommandée, il est vraisemblable qu'il ne s'accumulera pas dans l'environnement à des concentrations susceptibles de poser un problème écologique et il est improbable qu'il puisse avoir des effets nocifs sur les organismes terrestres et aquatiques.

3. Recommandations

- Les opérations de remplissage et l'épandage du 1,3-dichloropropène doivent obligatoirement s'accompagner des mesures de sécurité appropriées afin de faire en sorte que l'exposition ne dépasse pas les concentrations maximales autorisées.

- Il faudrait étudier la destinée métabolique du *trans*-1,3-dichloropropène chez les mammifères ainsi que le rôle que pourraient avoir les métabolites d'oxydation de cet isomère dans la toxicité du composé.

- L'effet protecteur du glutathion vis-à-vis du 1,3-dichloropropène est dû à l'action de la glutathion-transférase. Il est donc recommandé de procéder à des études afin de comparer la cinétique de l'action enzymatique de la glutathion-*S*-transférase humaine provenant des divers tissus à l'activité de l'enzyme d'origine animale provenant des tissus correspondants.

- Il conviendrait de rassembler et de publier les données dont on dispose sur le rôle protecteur du glutathion.

- La génotoxicité du dichloropropène est due pour une part à son métabolisme oxydatif. Il est recommandé d'entreprendre des études pour identifier l'isoenzyme responsable et la comparer à l'activité des isoenzymes du cytochrome P-450 humain.

- Dans les études de cancérogénicité où l'on procède par gavage des animaux, il conviendrait d'élucider le rôle de l'épichlorhydrine en tant que facteur de confusion éventuel.

RESUME ET EVALUATION, CONCLUSIONS, ET RECOMMANDATIONS
1,2-DICHLOROPROPANE

1. Résumé et évaluation

1.1 Usage, destinée et concentrations dans l'environnement

Le 1,2-dichloropropane est un liquide dont le point d'ébullition est de 96,8 °C et la tension de vapeur de 42 mmHg à 20 °C. Il est soluble dans l'eau, l'éthanol et l'éther éthylique. Par chauffage, il émet des vapeurs de phosgène hautement toxiques. Son coefficient de partage entre l'octanol et l'eau (log K_{ow}) est égal à 2,28.

Ce produit entre dans la composition des vernis pour meubles, des liquides de nettoyage à sec, des décapants pour peintures, des produits pour le dégraissage des surfaces métalliques, le traitement des huiles; il sert à la fabrication de caoutchoucs et de cires, ainsi que comme intermédiaire dans la production du tétrachloréthylène et du tétrachlorure de carbone. Il entre également dans la composition du mélange appelé D/D que l'on utilise comme fumigant avant la plantation.

Les mesures de la concentration du 1,2-dichloropropane dans l'air urbain ont donné des valeurs respectives de 1,2 $\mu g/m^3$ (valeur moyenne), 0,021-0,040 $\mu g/m^3$ et 0,0065-1,4 $\mu g/m^3$ respectivement à Philadelphie, Portland et au Japon. La décomposition dans l'atmosphère est lente; sur la base de la réaction avec les radicaux hydroxyles, on a évalué le temps de demi-décomposition du 1,2-dichloropropane à plus de 313 jours. Il est probable que la décomposition est essentiellement de nature photochimique. Pour que cette décomposition photochimique soit appréciable, il est nécessaire que le composé soit adsorbé sur des particules. C'est, semble-t-il, principalement par volatilisation que le 1,2-dichloropropane s'élimine de l'eau.

Dans le sol, les principales voies d'élimination sont la volatilisation et la diffusion. Le 1,2-dichloropropane persiste dans le sol. Plus de 98% du 1,2-dichloropropane appliqué sur du terreau ont été récupérés 12 à 20 semaines après ce traitement.

Il peut y avoir lessivage du 1,2-dichloropropane présent dans le sol et contamination des eaux souterraines à faible ou grande profondeur dans les secteurs traités avec des fumigants du type

"MIX D/D". Aux Etats-Unis d'Amérique, on a trouvé des concentrations dans l'eau de puits et les eaux souterraines allant respectivement jusqu'à 440 µg/litre et 51 µg/litre. Aux Pays-Bas, des concentrations atteignant 160 µg/litre ont été observées dans l'eau de puits et on a retrouvé du 1,2-dichloropropane jusqu'à une profondeur de 13 mètres.

Les plantes vivrières peuvent fixer le 1,2-dichloropropane mais les résidus qu'on y a décelés sont faibles (< 0,01 mg/kg) et probablement sans conséquence biologique.

La bioaccumulation du 1,2-dichloropropane est improbable en raison de sa forte solubilité dans l'eau (2,7 g/kg) et de la faible valeur de son coefficient de partage entre l'octanol et l'eau (log K_{ow}).

1.2 Cinétique et métabolisme

Administré par voie orale à des rats, le 1,2-dichloropropane est rapidement éliminé (80 à 90% en 24 h). Il n'y a pas de différences majeures dans la cinétique ou dans l'élimination entre les mâles et les femelles. La principale voie d'élimination est la voie urinaire, et jusqu'à la moitié de la dose orale initiale est éliminée dans les 24 h. La proportion éliminée par la voie fécale est inférieure à 10%. Le 1,2-dichloropropane est éliminé à hauteur de 33% dans l'air expiré, à la fois sous forme de dioxyde de carbone et d'un mélange de produits volatils. Les concentrations tissulaires sont faibles, la plus élevée étant observée au niveau du foie. Après exposition de rats par la voie respiratoire on note une élimination rapide du 1,2-dichloropropane; 55 à 65% de la dose initiale sont éliminés dans les urines et 16 à 23% dans l'air expiré. La demi-vie d'élimination à partir du sang est de 24 à 30 minutes.

On ne retrouve pas le 1,2-dichloropropane initial dans les urines. On y a identifié trois métabolites principaux. Ces métabolites résultent de l'oxydation et de la conjugaison du composé et aboutissent à la formation de mercapturates, de N-acétyl-S-(2-hydroxypropyl)-L-cystéine, de N-acétyl-S-(2-oxypropyl)-L-cystéine et de N-acétyl-S-(1-carboxyéthyl)-L-cystéine. Le 1,2-dichloropropane peut également subir une oxydation en lactate avec production de dioxyde de carbone ou d'acétyl-coenzyme A.

Après administration de 1,2-dichloropropane par voie orale à des rats à raison de 2 mg/kg, on a constaté une forte diminution du glutathion tissulaire. Il y avait également corrélation entre la diminution du glutathion tissulaire et les manifestations toxiques au niveau du foie, des reins et des hématies. Une réduction préalable du glutathion intracellulaire a provoqué une exacerbation de la toxicité du 1,2-dichloropropane, alors qu'un traitement préalable par des précurseurs de la synthèse du glutathion réduisait cette toxicité. Ces résultats montrent que le glutathion a un effet protecteur vis-à-vis des propriétés toxiques du 1,2-dichloropropane.

1.3 Effets sur les êtres vivant dans leur milieu naturel

On n'a pas déterminé la CE_{50} pour les algues d'eau douce car la volatilisation du composé à partir de la solution d'épreuve rend cette détermination difficile. La toxicité aiguë du 1,2-dichloropropane pour les invertébrés aquatiques et les poissons est faible à modérée; pour les invertébrés, les valeurs de la CL_{50} à 48 h varient de 52 à > 100 mg/litre, tandis que la CL50 à 96 h pour les poissons se situe entre 61 et 320 mg/litre. Une épreuve de toxicité à court terme effectuée sur des vairons du genre *Pimephales promelas* a montré que la dose maximale sans effet était de 82 mg/litre. Lors d'une épreuve de 32 jours sur les larves de ce vairon, on a constaté que les paramètres biologiques les plus sensibles à la toxicité du 1,2-dichloropropane étaient la croissance des larves et leur survie. On estime que la concentration maximale acceptable de substance toxique est de 6 à 11 mg/litre. Chez des poissons du genre *Pimelometopon* on a constaté une inhibition de la croissance après exposition de 33 jours à une concentration de 164 mg/litre.

Le 1,2-dichloropropane est phytotoxique.

Des épreuves par contact effectuées sur quatre espèces de lombrics ont montré que la CL_{50} se situait entre 44 et 84 $\mu g/cm^2$ (valeur moyenne) de papier filtre. Sur sol artificiel, les valeurs de la CL_{50} oscillaient entre 3880 et 5300 mg/kg de sol (en poids sec).

1.4 Effets sur les animaux d'expérience et les systèmes d'épreuve in vitro

Chez les animaux d'expérience, la toxicité aiguë par voie orale de ce composé est faible. Ainsi, la DL_{50} par voie orale est de 1,9 g/kg de poids corporel pour le rat et la DL_{50} cutanée est de 8,75 mg/kg de poids corporel chez le lapin.

Des études de toxicité de courte durée comportant l'administration de 1,2-dichloropropane par voie orale à des souris et à des rats ont montré qu'à des doses quotidiennes égales ou supérieures à 250 mg/kg de poids corporel, il y avait inhibition de la croissance, apparition de signes cliniques d'intoxication correspondant à une dépression du système nerveux central et accroissement de la mortalité. A la dose quotidienne de 250 mg/kg pendant dix jours, on a noté chez des rats une modification des enzymes sériques trahissant une légère hépatotoxicité, la dose sans effet observable étant de 100 mg/kg par jour.

Lors d'une étude par inhalation de 13 semaines effectuée sur des souris (à la dose maximale de 681 mg/m^3), on n'a pas observé d'effets nocifs. Lors d'une étude analogue sur des rats exposés à des doses de 68,1, 227 et 681 mg/m^3, on a observé une réduction du poids corporel et des lésions mineures du tissu des fosses nasales dans les groupes soumis aux deux plus fortes doses.

Lors d'une étude de reproduction portant sur deux générations de rats, on a donné aux animaux une eau de boisson contenant des concentrations de 1,2-dichloropropane respectivement égales à 0,024, 0,1, 0,24% (soit l'équivalent de 33,6, 140 et 336 mg/kg de poids corporel par jour); il en est résulté une réduction du gain de poids maternel et une diminution de la consommation d'eau, à la dose médiane et à la plus forte dose. Chez les animaux nouveaunés, le poids corporel était réduit à la dose la plus forte. La dose sans effet nocif observable s'établissait respectivement à 33,6 et 140 mg/kg de poids corporel par jour pour les effets toxiques sur la mère et sur la fonction de reproduction.

Les études ne mettent en évidence aucune activité tératogène du 1,2-dichloropropane à des doses orales allant jusqu'à 125 mg/kg de poids corporel chez le rat et 150 mg/kg de poids corporel chez le lapin. Toutefois à ces doses, on a observé une toxicité du produit pour les mères et pour les foetus, à en juger d'après certains signes cliniques témoignant d'une atteinte du système nerveux central, la réduction du gain de poids maternel et, chez les foetus, un retard d'ossification. La dose sans effet observable est égale à 30 mg/kg de poids corporel par jour chez le rat et à 50 mg/kg de poids corporel par jour chez le lapin.

La plupart des études ont mis en évidence une mutagénicité du 1,2-dichloropropane chez les bactéries avec ou sans activation métabolique, mais il est vrai qu'on avait utilisé des doses extrêmement élevées (jusqu'à 10 mg/boîte). Le 1,2-dichloropropane provoque des aberrations chromosomiques et des échanges entre chromatides soeurs dans les cellules ovariennes de hamster chinois; il y a également accroissement des échanges entre chromatides soeurs dans des cellules V79 de hamster chinois en présence de 1,2-dichloropropane. Des lymphocytes humains ont été cultivés en présence ou en l'absence d'un système métabolisant de foie de rat; on a constaté que ces cellules fixaient la thymidine tritiée de la même manière que les cultures témoins et qu'elles présentaient la même viabilité. Une épreuve de mutation létale récessive liée au sexe effectuée sur *Drosophila melanogaster* a donné des résultats négatifs. Une épreuve de létalité dominante chez des rats soumis pendant 14 semaines à des doses de 1,2-dichloropropane mêlé à leur eau de boisson, puis accouplés au cours des deux semaines suivantes, a donné des résultats également négatifs.

Lors d'une étude de cancérogénicité effectuée sur des souris, on a administré aux animaux par gavage, 125 ou 250 mg de 1,2-dichloropropane par kg de poids corporel; on a observé une augmentation, liée à la dose, de l'incidence des adénomes hépatiques. L'incidence des adénomes était plus élevée dans les groupes traités que dans le groupe témoin mais elle se situait malgré tout dans les limites normales pour les témoins historiques.

Chez des rats soumis à des doses de 125 et de 250 mg/kg de poids corporel (femelles) ou 62 et 125 mg/kg de poids corporel (mâles) par gavage, cinq jours par semaines pendant 113 semaines, on a noté une légère augmentation dans l'incidence des adénocarcinomes mammaires chez les femelles soumises à la dose la plus forte, augmentation qui était supérieure aux limites normales pour les témoins historique.

1.5 Effets sur l'homme

Il est improbable que la population générale soit exposée au 1,2-dichloropropane par l'intermédiaire de l'air et de l'eau, sauf dans les zones où l'on utilise largement le 1,2-dichloropropoane ou le "D/D MIX" à des fins agricoles. Les résidus de 1,2-dichloropropane présents dans les plantes vivrières sont généralement inférieurs à la limite de détection. L'exposition étant faible, on peut considérer que le risque est négligeable pour la population générale.

On a signalé plusieurs cas d'intoxication aiguë accidentelle ou intentionnelle (suicide) dus à une surexposition au 1,2-dichloropropane. Les effets en étaient essentiellement observables au niveau du système nerveux central, du foie et des reins. On a également fait état d'une anémie hémolytique et d'une coagulation intravasculaire disséminée. Dans un cas, le malade se trouvait dans un état de délire qui a évolué vers un état de choc irréversible et une insuffisance cardiaque fatale.

Il peut y avoir exposition professionnelle par voie cutanée ou respiratoire. On a fait état de plusieurs cas de dermatite ou de sensibilisation cutanée chez des travailleurs qui utilisaient des solvants contenant du 1,2-dichloropropane.

2. Conclusions

- Population générale: L'exposition de la population générale au 1,2-dichloropropane à partir de l'air ou de la nourriture est faible, voire inexistante. Toutefois dans certains secteurs, il peut y avoir exposition en cas de contamination des eaux souterraines.

- Exposition professionnelle: Moyennant de bonnes méthodes de travail et des précautions d'hygiène et de sécurité, il est peu probable que l'utilisation du 1,2-dichloropropane comporte un risque pour les personnes qui y sont exposées de par leur profession.

- Environnement: Il est improbable que le 1,2-dichloropropane s'accumule dans l'environnement à des concentrations écologiquement nocives lorsqu'on l'utilise à la dose recommandée. Il est également improbable qu'il produise des effets nocifs sur les populations d'organismes terrestres ou aquatiques.

3. Recommandations

- Il faudrait évaluer la toxicité aiguë par voie respiratoire ainsi que le pouvoir irritant pour les yeux et la peau et le pouvoir sensibilisant cutané de ce composé.

- Lorsqu'on manipule du 1,2-dichloropropane il faut prendre des mesures de sécurité appropriées afin d'éviter toute exposition supérieure à la concentration maximale admissible.

RESUME ET EVALUATION, CONCLUSIONS, ET RECOMMANDATIONS
"MIX D/D"

1. Résumé et évaluation

1.1 Usage, destinée et concentrations dans l'environnement

Le mélange technique de dichloropropènes et de dichloropropane (désignés dans la suite du texte par l'abréviation "MIX D/D") est un liquide limpide de couleur ambrée doté d'une odeur piquante; sa tension de vapeur est de 35 mmHg à 20 °C et il est soluble dans les solvants halogénés, les esters et les cétones.

Le MIX D/D présente une composition caractéristique, à savoir: au moins 50% de 1,3-dichloropropènes (proportion des isomères *cis*- et *trans*-, environ 1/1), les autres constituants principaux étant le 1,2-dichloropropane et les composés voisins. On l'a beaucoup utilisé comme nématocide en application sur le sol avant la plantation.

Le transport, la distribution et la destinée des principaux constituants du MIX D/D dans l'air, l'eau et le sol sont décrits à la section 4 des chapitres consacrées au 1,3-dichloropropène et au 1,2-dichloropropane.

Le 1,2-dichloropropane provenant du MIX D/D présent dans le sol a une certaine tendance à contaminer l'eau des puits et les eaux souterraines en général, par suite d'un phénomène de lessivage. Lors d'une opération de forage à des fins d'irrigation en Europe occidentale (68 m de profondeur) on a constaté que les concentrations moyennes de 1,2-dichloropropane à différentes profondeurs variaient entre 0,8 et 8,5 μg/litre, la concentration la plus élevée étant de 165 μg/litre.

Il est peu probable que les cultures fixent en proportion importante les constituants du MIX D/D (voir les autres chapitres de la présente monographie). Il est également peu probable que ces constituants subissent une bioaccumulation du fait que leur coefficient de partage entre l'octanol et l'eau (log K_{ow}) est faible et que leur solubilité dans l'eau est relativement forte.

1.2 Cinétique et métabolisme

On n'a pas procédé à des études métaboliques sur le MIX D/D. Les deux principaux constituants, le 1,3-dichloropropène et le 1,2-

dichloropropane sont rapidement éliminés, essentiellement dans l'urine et en moindre proportion, dans l'air expiré. Les constituants du MIX D/D sont métabolisés selon un processus qui comporte une oxydation et une conjugaison. Les principaux métabolites urinaires sont des acides mercapturiques.

1.3 Effets sur les organismes vivants dans leur milieu naturel

Le MIX D/D est modérément toxique pour les poissons; les valeurs de la CL_{50} à 96 h varient de 1 à 6 mg/litre. La toxicité du MIX D/D est largement imputable au 1,3-dichloropropène.

Lorsqu'on utilise ce mélange aux doses recommandées, ses effets principaux consistent dans une diminution passagère (moins de sept jours) des populations de champignons terricoles et une inhibition de l'oxydation de ions ammonium en nitrates. Le MIX D/D est toxique pour les bactéries nitrifiantes. Peu après la disparition du MIX D/D, le sol est recolonisé par les bactéries. Lors d'essais en situation réelle, on a constaté que le MIX D/D, appliqué à raison de 600 litres/hectare, provoquait la destruction des invertébrés terricoles. Il faut de 6 à 24 mois pour que la recolonisation s'effectue.

Le MIX D/D est extrêmement phytotoxique.

1.4 Effets sur les animaux d'expérience et les systèmes d'épreuve in vitro

Le MIX D/D présente une toxicité aiguë modérée à forte pour les animaux de laboratoire. Chez le rat et la souris, la DL_{50} par voie orale varie de 132 à 300 mg/kg de poids corporel. En ce qui concerne la DL_{50} par voie cutanée, les valeurs pour le rat et le lapin sont respectivement de 779 et de 2100 mg/kg de poids corporel. Chez le rat, la CL_{50} à 4 h par inhalation est approximativement égale à 4540 mg/m^3. En cas d'exposition, les signes cliniques observés sont ceux d'une dépression du système nerveux central. Le MIX D/D est fortement irritant pour les yeux et la peau et il est doté d'un pouvoir sensibilisateur cutané modéré.

Les résultats des études toxicologiques à court terme effectuées sur des rats et des chiens sont insuffisants pour qu'on puisse déterminer convenablement la toxicité du MIX D/D, car aux doses relativement faibles que l'on a étudiées, on n'observe pas d'effets biologiquement significatifs. Plusieurs études d'inhalation de courte durée (corps entier) ont été effectuées sur des rats. A des doses allant jusqu'à 145 mg/m^3, le MIX D/D n'a pas produit d'effets toxiques. A partir de 1362 mg/m^3, les effets toxiques étaient évidents et correspondaient à une dépression du système nerveux central. L'exposition des animaux à la dose de 443 mg/m^3 pendant 10 semaines a entraîné une réduction du gain de poids et une augmentation du poids des reins.

Une étude tératologique comportant l'administration de MIX D/D par voie orale n'a pas permis, en raison de ses insuffisances, d'évaluer le pouvoir tératogène de ce composé chez le rat.

Lors d'une étude d'inhalation chez le rat destinée à étudier les effets du MIX D/D sur la fécondité des mâles et des femelles, on n'a pas observé d'effets à des doses allant jusqu' 443 mg/m^3 sur une durée de dix semaines. Il n'a pas été possible de procéder à une évaluation complète des effets du MIX D/D sur la reproduction, en raison du caractère incomplet du protocole de ces études.

Le MIX D/D s'est révélé mutagène pour les souches TA100 et TA1535 de *Salmonella typhimurium* ainsi que pour la souche WP2 HCR d'*Escherichia coli*, sans activation métabolique. Cet effet n'a pas été observé sur les souches TA98, TA1537 et TA1538 de salmonelles.

Lors d'une étude à long terme, au cours de laquelle on avait administré à des rats un régime alimentaire contenant jusqu'à 120 mg/kg (soit 6 mg/kg de poids corporel) pendant deux ans, on n'a pas observé d'effets toxiques ou cancérogènes.

1.5 Effets sur l'homme

Le MIX D/D n'est plus guère utilisé et par conséquent il est peu probable que la population générale puisse être exposée par l'intermédiaire de l'air, de l'eau et des aliments. L'exposition des personnels qui remplissent les fûts ou qui sont chargés de l'épandage du produit s'est en général située en-dessous de 4,5 mg de 1,3-dichloropropène/m^3 lorsque l'on respectait la marche à suivre recommandée; dans d'autres cas, on a mesuré des concentrations allant jusqu'à 36,32 mg/m^3.

On a cité un cas d'intoxication aiguë mortelle par suite de l'ingestion accidentelle de MIX D/D.

2. Conclusions

- Population générale. Etant donné que l'on l'utilise plus guère le MIX D/D, l'exposition de la population générale au 1,3-dichloropropène par l'intermédiaire de l'air, de l'eau et des aliments est négligeable, mais dans certaines zones, il peut y avoir exposition au 1,2-dichloropropane en cas de contamination des eaux souterraines.

- Exposition professionnelle. Lors du remplissage des fûts et de l'épandage du MIX D/D, il peut y avoir exposition des personnels concernés au 1,3-dichloropropène, à des concentrations qui dépassent les valeurs maximales admissibles, en particulier sous les climats chauds.

- Environnement. Il est peu probable que le MIX D/D atteigne dans l'environnement des concentrations biologiquement nocives pour la faune et la flore terrestre ou aquatique, lorsqu'on utilise la dose recommandée. Il est également improbable qu'il puisse exercer des effets nocifs durables sur les organismes vivants dans leur milieu naturel.

3. Recommandations

- Le MIX D/D ne doit pas être utilisé comme fumigant pour traiter le sol du fait qu'il risque de passer dans les eaux souterraines par lessivage.

- Dans les zones où l'on a utilisé du MIX D/D, il faut surveiller les eaux de surface et les eaux souterraines à la recherche de résidus éventuels.

RESUMEN Y EVALUACION, CONCLUSIONES, Y RECOMENDACIONES
1,3-DICLOROPROPENO

1. Resumen y evaluación

1.1 Uso, destino y niveles en el medio ambiente

El "1,3-dicloropropeno" se introdujo en 1956 como parte de una mezcla, que contenía 1,3-dicloropropeno, 1,2-dicloropropano y otros hidrocarburos halogenados, y se ha utilizado ampliamente en la agricultura como fumigante del suelo que se destina a nuevas plantaciones para combatir los nematodos de las hortalizas, las papas y el tabaco. Se aplica fundamentalmente mediante inyección en el suelo. La formulación comercial del 1,3-dicloropropeno es una mezcla de isómeros *cis* y *trans* (aproximadamente en proporciones iguales), que forman un líquido entre incoloro y ámbar, con un olor penetrante e irritante, parecido al del cloroformo. La presión del vapor es de 3,7 kPa a 20 °C. El producto técnico tiene una pureza del 92% y puede contener varias impurezas, como 1,2-dicloropropano. El log P del coeficiente de reparto octanol/agua es de 1,98.

En el aire, la descomposición del 1,3-dicloropropeno tiene lugar sobre todo por reacción con radicales libres y con el ozono. La semivida de los isómeros *cis* y *trans* en la reacción con radicales libres es de 12 y 7 horas respectivamente, y en la reacción con el ozono de 52 y 12 días respectivamente. La fototransformación directa parece ser insignificante, pero puede aumentar en presencia de partículas atmosféricas.

En el agua, el 1,3-dicloropropeno tiende a desaparecer con rapidez, debido a su solubilidad relativamente baja en ella y su elevada volatilidad; se han notificado semividas de menos de 5 h.

La distribución del 1,3-dicloropropeno en los compartimentos del suelo depende de la presión del vapor, el coeficiente de difusión, la temperatura y el contenido de humedad del mismo. En la persistencia del 1,3-dicloropropeno en el suelo influyen la volatilización, la transformación química y biológica, la transformación fotoquímica y la absorción por los organismos. Los mecanismos más importantes de dispersión y dilución en el medio ambiente son la volatilización y la difusión en la fase de vapor.

La transformación del 1,3-dicloropropeno se produce inicialmente por hidrólisis a 3-cloroalilalcohol y luego por transformación microbiana a 3-cloroacroleína y ácido 3-cloroacrílico. En un estudio de laboratorio, la semivida de la hidrólisis de los isómeros *cis* y *trans* del 1,3-dicloropropeno a 15 °C y 29 °C fue de 11,0 y 2,0 días respectivamente para el isómero *cis* y de 13,0 y 2,0 días para el isómero *trans*. En el suelo, con un pH 7 y una temperatura de 25 °C, la semivida de la hidrólisis fue de 4,6 días para ambos isómeros. Debido a su desaparición relativamente rápida del suelo, no es probable que se acumulen residuos cuando se aplica el fumigante con la dosis y la frecuencia recomendadas.

El 1,3-dicloropropeno puede desplazarse en el suelo, sobre todo si es arenoso, de textura gruesa y con un contenido bajo de humedad. El desplazamiento descendente se ve favorecido por el cultivo profundo de los suelos con escasa porosidad. Se ha detectado 1,3-dicloropropeno en "aguas subterráneas altas" (hasta 2 m por debajo de la superficie), pero no en las profundas, que son las que suelen utilizarse para beber.

Los cultivos pueden absorber 1,3-dicloropropeno. Sin embargo, no es probable que aparezca una cantidad apreciable de residuos en las plantas cultivadas comestibles, que se suelen sembrar cuando ya ha desaparecido la mayor parte del fumigante.

Es poco probable la bioacumulación de 1,3-dicloropropeno, debido a su solubilidad relativamente alta en agua (< 1 g/kg), al bajo log P del coeficiente de reparto octanol/agua y a la eliminación rápida en mamíferos y otros organismos.

1.2 Cinética y metabolismo

El 1,3-dicloropropeno se elimina rápidamente tras su administración oral a roedores. La principal vía de eliminación es la orina, donde a ella el 81% de los isómeros *cis* y el 56% de los *trans* se eliminan en las 24 horas siguientes a la dosificación. La semivida de la eliminación en la orina es de 5 a 6 horas. La eliminación fecal es escasa. El anhídrido carbónico representa el 4 y el 24%, respectivamente, de los isómeros *cis* y *trans* del 1,3-dicloropropeno eliminados. Las concentraciones en los tejidos tras la administración oral son bajas; los niveles residuales más elevados se encuentran en la pared estomacal, seguidos por cantidades más bajas en los riñones y la vejiga.

1,3-Dichloropropene

No se ha detectado en la orina la presencia de 1,3-dicloropropeno inalterado. La glutatión-*S*-alquiltransferasa actúa sobre los isómeros *cis* y *trans* formando ácidos mercaptúricos, que se excretan por la orina. El isómero *trans* se conjuga de 4 a 5 veces más lentamente que el *cis*. El principal metabolito urinario en ratas y ratones es la *N*-acetil-*S*-(3-cloroprop-2-enil)L-cisteína; este metabolito se puede utilizar para la vigilancia biológica en el ser humano. Para el isómero *cis* se ha identificado una segunda ruta metabólica de menor importancia, en la que se produce una monooxigenación a óxido de *cis*-1,3-dicloropropeno, que se puede conjugar también con el glutatión. La elevada proporción del isómero *trans* que se encuentra en el aire expirado procede de una ruta metabólica distinta de la conjugación, que tiene una especificidad más elevada para el isómero *trans* que para el *cis*.

La exposición de ratas al 1,3-dicloropropeno por inhalación no produce un aumento de la concentración en sangre proporcional a la dosis. A una dosis de 408,6 mg/m^3 (90 ppm), disminuyeron la frecuencia respiratoria y el volumen respiratorio por minuto, y la saturación del metabolismo se produjo a 1362 mg/m^3 (300 ppm). Los isómeros *cis* y *trans* se eliminaron rápidamente de la sangre, siendo la semivida de la eliminación de 3 a 6 minutos para concentraciones inferiores a 1362 mg/m^3, pero considerablemente más larga (33-43 min.) a concentraciones más elevadas.

1.3 Efectos en los seres vivos del medio ambiente

Los valores de la CE_{50} para el crecimiento (96 h) del alga de agua dulce *Selenastrum capricornutum* y la diatomea de los estuarios *Skeletoneria costatum* son 4,95 mg/litro y 1 mg/litro respectivamente. La toxicidad aguda (CL_{50} a las 96 h) del 1,3-dicloropropeno para los peces es del orden de 1 a 7,9 mg/litro. En una prueba en embriones-larvas de *Pimephales promelas*, el nivel máximo sin efectos fue de 0,24 mg/litro. Estos datos, junto con el hecho de que no es probable que el 1,3-dicloropropeno persista en el agua, indican que el peligro para los peces lo constituyen los efectos tóxicos agudos, con escasas posibilidades de efectos adicionales debidos a la exposición durante un tiempo prolongado.

En dosis de 30 a 60 mg/kg, el 1,3-dicloropropeno puede reducir la concentración de hongos y la tasa de actividad enzimática microbiana, pero el efecto no suele ser duradero (< 7 días) y no se produce en todos los tipos de suelos. En algunos estudios, aumentó significativamente el número de microorganismos tras la aplicación.

El 1,3-dicloropropeno es fitotóxico, pero su toxicidad para las abejas es escasa. Utilizando una técnica de espolvoreo, la DL_{50} a las 48 horas fue de 6,6 µg/abeja. Las aves tienen una sensibilidad relativamente baja al 1,3-dicloropropeno. Para el pato real (*Anas platyrhynchos*) y la codorniz (*Colinus virginianus*) se ha informado de CL_{50} (8 días) de > 10 g/kg de la dieta.

1.4 Efectos en los animales de experimentación y en sistemas de prueba in vitro

La toxicidad aguda por vía oral del 1,3-dicloropropeno en animales es de moderada a alta. Se han notificado valores de la DL_{50} en ratas que oscilan entre 127 y 713 mg/kg de peso corporal. Los valores de la DL_{50} por vía oral en ratas para los isómeros *cis* y *trans* fueron de 85 y 94 mg/kg de peso corporal, respectivamente.

La exposición aguda cutánea es moderadamente tóxica. En ratas y conejos se ha reportado de una DL_{50} de 423 mg/kg y 504 mg/kg de peso corporal, respectivamente. Los valores de la DL_{50} para los isómeros *cis* y *trans* fueron 1090 y 1575 mg/kg de peso corporal, respectivamente.

La exposición por inhalación (4 h) en ratas dio como resultado valores de la DL_{50} de 3310 mg/m^3 (729 ppm) para el 1,3-dicloropropeno; 3042 mg/m^3 -3514 mg/m^3 para el isómero *cis* y 4880 mg/m^3 - 5403 mg/m^3 para el *trans*.

La intoxicación aguda afectó el sistema nervioso central y el aparato respiratorio.

En pruebas cutáneas y de irritación ocular con conejos se observaron reacciones graves, pero la recuperación se produjo en un período de 14-21 días. Los resultados de las pruebas de sensibilización en cobayos fueron positivos.

Se han realizado varios estudios de toxicidad por inhalación durante un tiempo breve en ratones, ratas, cobayos, conejos y perros. En los ratones los órganos afectados fueron la mucosa nasal y la vejiga urinaria. Se observó degeneración del epitelio olfatorio e hiperplasia del epitelio respiratorio. Se detectó hiperplasia del epitelio de transición de la vejiga urinaria. En ratones se puede estimar que el nivel sin efectos observados (NOEL) es de 136 mg/m^3 (30 ppm).

En ratas también se han detectado cambios degenerativos similares en el epitelio olfatorio, así como hiperplasia. En un estudio bien diseñado se encontró un valor del NOEL para el 1,3-dicloropropeno de 45,4 mg/m^3, siendo el valor del NOEL para el isómero *cis* de 136 mg/m^3.

En un estudio de administración por vía oral durante 90 días a ratas, el NOEL fue de 3 mg/kg de peso corporal. El único efecto observado con la dosis inmediatamente superior, de 10 mg/kg de peso corporal, fue un aumento relativo del peso de los riñones en los machos.

En un estudio de inhalación sobre la reproducción de dos camadas en dos generaciones de ratas, las dosis de hasta 408,6 mg/m^3 (90 ppm) no produjeron efectos adversos sobre los parámetros de la reproducción examinados. Sin embargo, la dosis más alta, de 408,6 mg/m^3, indujo toxicidad materna, que se puso de manifiesto por la disminución del crecimiento y por cambios histopatológicos de la mucosa nasal. Se estableció un NOEL para la toxicidad materna de 136,2 mg/m^3 (30 ppm).

En estudios de teratogenicidad por inhalación en ratas y conejos, el 1,3-dicloropropeno no mostró potencial teratogénico a niveles de exposición de hasta 1362 mg/m^3, pero se observó embriotoxicidad (reducción del tamaño de la camada y aumento del índice de reabsorciones) en ratas. Con dosis de 544,8 mg/m^3 (120 ppm) o superiores se advirtió toxicidad materna tanto en ratas como en conejos.

En la mayor parte de los estudios, el 1,3-dicloropropeno *cis* y *trans* y la mezcla de ambos fueron mutagénicos en bacterias, con y sin activación metabólica. Se encontró que el 1,3-dicloropropeno puro y el *cis*-1,3-dicloropropeno puro carecían de efecto sobre las bacterias. Se demostró que el glutatión impedía la actividad mutagénica del 1,3-dicloropropeno en bacterias. En un ensayo de mutación genética con células de hámster chino V79, así como en la prueba del locus HPRT de ovario de hámster chino, el *cis*-1,3-dicloropropeno dio un resultado negativo.

El 1,3-dicloropropeno *cis* y *trans* indujo una síntesis no programada de ADN en células S_3 HeLa. En hepatocitos de rata, el 1,3-dicloropropeno no produjo una reparación significativa del ADN. En el ensayo del locus rec con microsomas de la cepa H17 de *Bacillus subtilis* con activación metabólica, el 1,3-dicloropropeno dio resultado positivo.

En células de ovario de hámster chino, el 1,3-dicloropropeno *cis* y *trans* indujo daños cromosómicos en condiciones de activación metabólica, pero en otro estudio también dio resultado positivo sin que hubiera activación. El isómero *cis* no indujo lesiones cromosómicas en células hepáticas de rata, pero sí un intercambio de cromátidas hermanas en células de ovario de hámster chino con activación metabólica y sin ella, y en células de hámster chino V79 sin activación.

En una prueba con micronúcleos de médula ósea en ratones, y en otra de letalidad recesiva ligada al sexo en *Drosophila melanogaster*, el 1,3-dicloropropeno fue negativo.

Se realizaron estudios de carcinogenicidad en ratones y ratas. Se administró 1,3-dicloropropeno de calidad técnica (con un 1% de epiclorhidrina) mediante sonda durante dos años. En los ratones se observó un aumento significativo de la hiperplasia epitelial y los carcinomas celulares transitorios en la vejiga urinaria, una incidencia mayor de tumores pulmonares, un ligero aumento de tumores hepáticos y una mayor proporción de hiperplasia epitelial y papilomas o carcinomas de las células escamosas de la parte cardíaca del estómago.

En estudios de inhalación de dos años se investigó la carcinogenicidad del 1,3-dicloropropeno (sin epiclorhidrina) en ratones y ratas. En ratones se detectó una mayor incidencia de hiperplasia en la vejiga urinaria, la parte cardíaca del estómago y la mucosa nasal. Aumentó la incidencia de los tumores pulmonares benignos. También se observaron en ratas algunos cambios tóxicos en la mucosa olfativa de la cavidad nasal, pero sin aumento de la incidencia de tumores.

En un estudio de administración con sonda se puso de manifiesto que la epiclorhidrina producía tumores en la parte cardíaca del estómago, y en otro estudio de inhalación en ratas aparecieron tumores en la cavidad nasal; en el caso de la administración de 1,3-dicloropropeno por vía oral a ratones no se puede excluir un efecto carcinogénico sobre la vejiga urinaria.

Mecanismo de acción

Dado que la principal ruta metabólica de eliminación del 1,3-dicloropropeno es mediante la conjugación con el glutatión, cabe esperar que las condiciones que alteran la concentración de glutatión (sulfhidrilo no proteico) en los tejidos puedan modificar los efectos del compuesto. El mismo 1,3-dicloropropeno agota el contenido de glutatión de diversos tejidos, especialmente los situados en puntos de entrada en el organismo, es decir, sobre todo la parte cardíaca del estómago y el hígado tras la administración con sonda y el tejido nasal después de la exposición por inhalación. Tras la inhalación de concentraciones de 1,3-dicloropropeno superiores a 22,7 mg/m^3 (5 ppm) y 113,5 mg/m^3 (25 ppm) se produjo, respectivamente, una disminución de los niveles de glutatión en el epitelio nasal y en la parte cardíaca del estómago en ratones.

La toxicidad del 1,3-dicloropropeno en animales se produce con niveles de exposiciones que agotan el glutatión de los tejidos y la disminución previa de la concentración de éste la agrava. La inhalación durante un tiempo prolongado de concentraciones superiores a 90,8 mg/m^3 (20 ppm) da lugar en ratones a degeneración e hiperplasia del epitelio nasal y gástrico, mientras que en ratas la inhalación durante un tiempo prolongado de una concentración de 272,4 mg/m^3 (60 ppm) produce degeneración del tejido nasal.

La función protectora del glutatión se ha puesto de relieve ulteriormente en estudios que han demostrado que la unión mediante enlaces covalentes del ^{14}C-1,3-dicloropropeno a la parte cardíaca del estómago de ratón aumentaba a medida que disminuía el contenido de sulfhidrilo no proteico. De igual forma, en sistemas de prueba *in vitro* el glutatión mejoró notablemente la genotoxicidad del 1,3-dicloropropeno y del óxido 1,3-dicloropropeno, su metabolito oxidativo secundario (citocromo P-450).

1.5 Efectos en el ser humano

No es probable la exposición de la población general a través del aire, el agua o los alimentos.

En los estudios realizados se ha puesto de manifiesto que la exposición profesional está en general por debajo de 4,54 mg/m^3 (1 ppm), pero también se han notificado niveles más elevados (hasta 18,3 mg/m^3 durante el llenado o el cambio de la boquilla). Es probable que la exposición profesional se produzca por inhalación y por vía cutánea. Tras la exposición aparece inmediatamente irritación de los ojos y de la parte superior de la mucosa respiratoria. La inhalación de aire con concentraciones de > 6810 mg/m^3 (> 1500 ppm) produjo signos y síntomas de intoxicación grave; las exposiciones más bajas dieron lugar a una depresión del sistema nervioso central y a la irritación del aparato respiratorio. La exposición cutánea produjo una irritación grave de la piel.

Se notificó que un grupo de aplicadores de 1,3-dicloropropeno tuvieron algunos cambios en las funciones renal y hepática al final de la temporada de aplicación. Sin embargo, se ha rebatido la relación causa-efecto.

Se han producido algunos casos de intoxicación con hospitalización de los afectados, que presentaban signos y síntomas de irritación de la membrana mucosa, malestar torácico, dolor de cabeza, náuseas, vómitos, mareos y, en ocasiones, pérdida del conocimiento y disminución de la libido. Se han atribuido tres casos de enfermedades malignas sanguíneas a una sobreexposición accidental anterior al 1,3-dicloropropeno, pero la relación causa-efecto sigue siendo dudosa.

Se comparó el estado de fecundidad de un grupo de personas que trabajaban en la producción de compuestos clorados de tres carbonos con otro testigo. No se demostró la existencia de una asociación entre la disminución de la fecundidad y la exposición.

2. Conclusiones

Población general: A la vista del grado de exposición bajo o nulo al 1,3-dicloropropeno, el riesgo para la población general es insignificante.

Exposición profesional: Cuando no se adoptan las precauciones adecuadas de seguridad, las actividades de llenado y aplicación en el campo pueden dar lugar a una exposición del operador a concentraciones que superan el máximo permisible.

Medio ambiente: Siempre que se utilice el 1,3-dicloropropeno en la proporción recomendada, no es probable que se alcancen niveles importantes para el medio ambiente, y tampoco es probable que produzca efectos secundarios sobre poblaciones de seres vivos terrestres y acuáticos.

3. Recomendaciones

- Las actividades de llenado y la aplicación en el campo del 1,3-dicloropropeno sólo deben realizarse tomando las precauciones de seguridad adecuadas, a fin de tener la garantía de que los niveles de exposición no exceden las concentraciones máximas permisibles de este producto.

- Se deben realizar estudios a fin de investigar el destino metabólico del isómero *trans* del 1,3-dicloropropeno en mamíferos y la posible función que los metabolitos oxidativos de este isómero pueden tener como intermediarios en la toxicidad del 1,3-dicloropropeno.

- La glutatión transferasa interviene en el efecto protector del glutatión frente a la toxicidad del 1,3-dicloropropeno. Se recomienda la realización de estudios que permitan comparar la cinética enzimática relativa de la glutatión S-transferasa humana de diversos tejidos con la actividad enzimática de tejidos animales comparables.

- Se deben agrupar y publicar en revistas con una difusión amplia los datos disponibles acerca de la función protectora del glutatión.

- Parte de la genotoxicidad del dicloropropeno se debe al metabolismo oxidativo. Se recomienda la realización de estudios para identificar la isoenzima del citocromo P-450 que lleva a cabo esta acción y comparar su actividad con la de las isoenzimas del citocromo P-450 humano.

- Hay que aclarar la confusa función de la epiclorhidrina en los estudios de carcinogenicidad por vía oral con sonda.

RESUMEN Y EVALUACION, CONCLUSIONES Y RECOMENDACIONES
1,2-DICLOROPROPANO

1. Resumen y evaluación

1.1 Uso, destino y niveles en el medio ambiente

El 1,2-dicloropropano es un líquido con un punto de ebullición de 96,8 °C y una presión del vapor de 42 mm de Hg a 20 °C. Es soluble en agua, etanol y éter etílico. Al calentarlo desprende vapores de fosgeno enormemente tóxicos. El log P del coeficiente de reparto octanol/agua es de 2,28.

Es una sustancia que se usa en el acabado de muebles, líquidos de limpieza en seco, decapantes para pinturas, tratamiento de la cola, desengrasado de metales, tratamiento del petróleo y como ingrediente en la fabricación de caucho y de cera y como producto químico intermedio en la fabricación de tetracloroetileno y tetracloruro de carbono. Forma parte de la mezcla D/D, utilizada como fumigante antes de la siembra.

Se han determinado las concentraciones de 1,2-dicloropropano en el aire de las ciudades, con 1,2 $\mu g/m^3$ (valor medio), 0,021-0,040 $\mu g/m^3$ y 0,0065-1,4 $\mu g/m^3$ en Filadelfia, Portland y Japón, respectivamente. Su descomposición en la atmósfera es lenta; en función de su reacción con los radicales oxhidrilos, la semivida del 1,2-dicloropropano fue de > 313 días. Probablemente el proceso predominante en su descomposición es la fototransformación. Para que ésta sea apreciable es necesario que haya adsorción sobre material particulado. Es probable que la volatilización sea la principal vía de escape del agua.

En el suelo, los principales mecanismos de eliminación son la volatilización y la difusión. El 1,2-dicloropropano es persistente en el suelo. Más del 98% del aplicado a suelos de marga se recuperó a las 12-20 semanas del tratamiento.

En zonas en las que se ha utilizado la "mezcla D/D" para fumigar el suelo, el 1,2-dicloropropano puede contaminar por lixiviación las aguas subterráneas altas y profundas. En los Estados Unidos se han encontrado en el agua de pozo y la subterránea concentraciones de hasta 440 μg/litro y 51 μg/litro, respectivamente. En los Países Bajos se han medido concentraciones de hasta 160 μg/litro en agua de pozo, y se ha encontrado 1,2-dicloropropano a una profundidad de 13 metros.

El 1,2-dicloropropano se puede ingerir con los cultivos comestibles, pero los residuos detectados eran bajos (< 0,01 mg/kg) y no parece que puedan tener significación biológica.

No es probable la bioacumulación de 1,2-dicloropropano, debido a su elevada solubilidad en agua (2,7 g/kg) y al bajo log P del coeficiente de reparto octanol/agua.

1.2 Cinética y metabolismo

El 1,2-dicloropropano administrado a ratas por vía oral se elimina rápidamente (80-90% en 24 horas). No existen grandes diferencias entre machos y hembras en cuanto a la cinética o la eliminación. La principal vía de eliminación es la orina, excretandose en 24 horas hasta la mitad de una dosis oral. Por las heces se elimina menos del 10%. Un tercio se expulsa en el aire expirado, en forma de anhídrido carbónico y como mezcla de productos volátiles. Las concentraciones en los tejidos son bajas, detectándose la más alta en el hígado. Tras la exposición de ratas por inhalación, también se produce una eliminación rápida; en la orina se expulsa el 55-65% de la dosis, y el 16-23% en el aire expirado. La semivida en la sangre es de 24-30 minutos.

No se ha encontrado en la orina 1,2-dicloropropano inalterado. Se han identificado tres metabolitos urinarios principales. Estos proceden de las vías oxidativa y de conjugación, que dan lugar a los mercapturatos, N-acetil-S-(2-hidroxipropil)-L-cisteína, N-acetil-S-(2-oxipropil)-L-cisteína y N-acetil-S-(1-carboxietil)-L-cisteína. El 1,2-dicloropropano también se puede oxidar a lactato y dar anhídrido carbónico o acetil-CoA como producto final.

La administración de 1,2-dicloropropano por vía oral a ratas (2 ml/kg) produjo una notable reducción de la concentración de glutatión en los tejidos. Había una correlación entre la pérdida de glutatión y las características de la toxicidad en el hígado, los riñones y los eritrocitos. La disminución previa del glutatión intracelular agravaba la toxicidad del 1,2-dicloropropano, mientras que un tratamiento anterior con precursores de la síntesis del glutatión mejoraba la toxicidad. Estos resultados demuestran el efecto protector del glutatión frente a la toxicidad del 1,2-dicloropropano.

1.3 Efectos en los seres vivos del medio ambiente

No se ha calculado la CE_{50} para las algas de agua dulce por las dificultades que plantea la volatilización del producto de la solución de prueba. La toxicidad aguda del 1,2-dicloropropano para los invertebrados acuáticos y los peces es de baja a moderada; los valores de la CL_{50} a las 48 h para los invertebrados oscila entre 52 y > 100 mg/litro, y para los peces a las 96 h varía entre 61 y 320 mg/litro. En las pruebas de toxicidad durante un período corto con *Pimephales promelas* se calculó un nivel máximo sin efectos observados de 82 mg/litro. En una prueba de toxicidad de 32 días en las primeras fases de vida de la misma especie se puso de manifiesto que el crecimiento y la supervivencia de las larvas eran los parámetros más sensibles. La máxima concentración tóxica aceptable (MCTA) se estimó entre 6 y 11 mg/litro. A los 33 días de exposición a concentraciones de 164 mg/litro de 1,2-dicloropropano se advirtió inhibición del crecimiento en *Cyprinodon variegatus*.

El 1,2-dicloropropano es fitotóxico.

En las pruebas de contacto con cuatro especies de lombrices de tierra se obtuvo una CL_{50} de 44-84 $\mu g/cm^2$ (valores medios) de papel de filtro. Los valores de la CL_{50} en suelo artificial fueron de 3880-5300 mg/kg de suelo (peso seco).

1.4 Efectos en los animales de experimentación y en sistemas de prueba in vitro

La toxicidad aguda por vía oral del 1,2-dicloropropano en animales de experimentación es baja. La DL_{50} por vía oral para la rata es de 1,9 g/kg de peso corporal, y por vía cutánea en conejos de 8,75 ml/kg de peso corporal.

En los estudios de toxicidad oral durante un período corto en ratones y ratas se puso de manifiesto una inhibición del crecimiento, signos clínicos de toxicidad asociados con una depresión del sistema nervioso central y/o un aumento de la mortalidad con dosis de 250 mg/kg de peso corporal al día o superiores. En ratas con una dosis diaria de 250 mg/kg de peso corporal durante 10 días se observaron cambios en las enzimas del suero que indicaban una ligera hepatotoxicidad, con un NOEL de 100 mg/kg al día.

En un estudio de inhalación durante 13 semanas en ratones (dosis máxima de 681 mg/m^3) no se observaron efectos adversos. En un estudio similar en el que se expusieron ratas a 68,1, 227 ó 681 mg/m^3, se produjo una disminución del peso corporal y ligeras lesiones en el tejido nasal en los grupos con las dos dosis más elevadas.

En un estudio de reproducción en dos generaciones, la exposición de ratas a proporciones de 1,2-dicloropropano en el agua de bebida del 0,024, el 0,1 y el 0,24% (equivalentes a 33,6, 140 y 336 mg/kg de peso corporal al día) dio lugar a un menor aumento del peso corporal en la madre y a un consumo reducido de agua con las dosis media y alta. El peso corporal de los recién nacidos fue menor con las dosis más altas. Se estableció un NOAEL para la toxicidad en las madres y en la reproducción de 33,6 y 140 mg/kg de peso corporal al día, respectivamente.

En los estudios realizados no se observó actividad teratogénica alguna del 1,2-dicloropropano con dosis orales de hasta 125 mg/kg de peso corporal en la rata y 150 mg/kg de peso corporal en el conejo. Sin embargo, a estas dosis el 1,2-dicloropropano era tóxico para las madres y los fetos, como pusieron de manifiesto los signos clínicos asociados al sistema nervioso central, el menor aumento del peso corporal de las madres y el retraso de la osificación en los fetos. Los NOEL son de 30 y 50 mg/kg de peso corporal al día para la rata y el conejo, respectivamente.

En la mayor parte de los estudios con bacterias, con activación metabólica o sin ella, el 1,2-dicloropropano mostró efectos mutagénicos, pero se utilizaron dosis muy elevadas, de hasta 10 mg/placa. En células de ovario de hámster chino se produjeron aberraciones cromosómicas e intercambio de cromátidas hermanas. En células V79 de hámster chino aumentó el intercambio de cromátidas. En un sistema *in vitro* con linfocitos humanos, la absorción de timidina tritiada y la viabilidad de las células cultivadas con un sistema metabolizante hepático de la rata y sin él fueron análogas a las de los cultivos testigo. Los resultados de una prueba de letalidad recesiva ligada al sexo en *Drosophila melanogaster* fueron negativos. En una prueba de letalidad dominante en ratas, en la que se administró el 1,2-dicloropropano con el agua de bebida durante 14 semanas, seguidas de dos semanas de apareamiento, se obtuvieron resultados negativos.

En un estudio de carcinogenicidad en ratones se administraron 125 ó 250 mg de 1,2-dicloropropano/kg de peso corporal mediante sonda, observándose un aumento relacionado con la dosis en la incidencia de adenomas hepáticos. Esta fue mayor en los grupos tratados que en el grupo testigo, pero se mantuvo dentro de los valores habituales de los testigos.

La administración por sonda en ratas, a concentraciones de 125 y 250 mg/kg de peso corporal (hembras) y 62 y 125 mg/kg de peso corporal (machos), cinco días a la semana durante 113 semanas, produjo en las hembras con la dosificación más alta un ligero aumento de la incidencia de adenocarcinomas de las glándulas mamarias, por encima de los valores habituales.

1.5 Efectos en el ser humano

No es probable la exposición de la población general al 1,2-dicloropropano a través del aire y el agua, excepto en zonas con un uso abundante de 1,2-dicloropropano y de mezcla D/D en la agricultura. Los residuos de 1,2-dicloropropano en los cultivos comestibles se suelen mantener por debajo del límite de detección. En vista de estos bajos niveles de exposición, el riesgo para la población general es insignificante.

Se han notificado varios casos de intoxicación aguda por 1,2-dicloropropano, debidos a una exposición excesiva accidental o intencionada (suicidio). Los efectos se han concentrado principalmente en el sistema nervioso central, el hígado y los riñones. También se ha descrito la aparición de anemia hemolítica y coagulación intravascular diseminada. En un caso, el delirio evolucionó hacia un shock irreversible, insuficiencia cardíaca y la muerte.

Se puede producir exposición profesional a través de la piel o por inhalación. Se ha informado de varios casos de dermatitis y de sensibilización cutánea en trabajadores que utilizaban mezclas de disolventes con 1,2-dicloropropano.

2. Conclusiones

- Población general: La exposición de la población general al 1,2-dicloropropano a partir del aire o los alimentos es baja o nula. Sin embargo, se puede producir en determinadas zonas una exposición debida a la contaminación de las aguas subterráneas.

- Exposición profesional: Con unas buenas prácticas de trabajo, medidas higiénicas y precauciones de seguridad, no es probable que el 1,2-dicloropropano represente un riesgo para las personas profesionalmente expuestas a él.

- Medio ambiente: Utilizado en las dosis recomendadas, no es probable que el 1,2-dicloropropano alcance niveles significativos en el medio ambiente. Tampoco es probable que tenga efectos adversos sobre las poblaciones de seres vivos terrestres y acuáticos.

3. Recomendaciones

- Se deben realizar estudios a fin de evaluar la toxicidad aguda por inhalación, la irritación ocular y cutánea y la posible sensibilización de la piel.

- Se han de adoptar las precauciones de seguridad apropiadas cuando se maneje 1,2-dicloropropano, a fin de evitar exposiciones que superen la concentración máxima permisible.

RESUMEN Y EVALUACION, CONCLUSIONES Y RECOMENDACIONES "MEZCLA D/D"

1. Resumen y evaluación

1.1 Uso, destino y niveles en el medio ambiente

La mezcla técnica de dicloropropenos y dicloropropano (abreviada en el presente texto como "mezcla D/D") es un líquido de color ámbar claro y olor acre; la presión del vapor es de 35 mm de Hg a 20 °C, y es soluble en disolventes halogenados, ésteres y cetonas.

La "mezcla D/D" suele contener no menos del 50% de 1,3-dicloropropeno (con isómeros *cis* y *trans* en una proporción aproximada de 1:1), y los demás ingredientes principales son el 1,2-dicloropropano y compuestos afines. Esta mezcla se utiliza mucho como nematocida del suelo antes de la siembra.

El transporte, la distribución y el destino en el medio ambiente de los componentes principales de la "mezcla D/D" en el aire, el agua y el suelo se describen en sección 4 de los apartados de la presente monografía de EHC que tratan del 1,3-dicloropropeno y el 1,2-dicloropropano.

El 1,2-dicloropropano procedente de la "mezcla D/D" tiene considerables posibilidades de escapar del suelo por lixiviación y contaminar las aguas de los pozos y las subterráneas. En un pozo de riego (68 m de profundidad) de Europa occidental se registraron unas concentraciones medias de 1,2-dicloropropano a diferentes profundidades que oscilaban entre 0,8 y 8,5 μg/litro, con una concentración máxima de 165 μg/litro.

No es probable que los cultivos absorban cantidades importantes de los componentes de la "mezcla D/D" (véase en otros apartados de la presente monografía). Tampoco es probable la bioacumulación de los componentes de la mezcla debido a su bajo log P del coeficiente de reparto octanol/agua y a su solubilidad relativamente grande en agua.

1.2 Cinética y metabolismo

No se han realizado estudios metabólicos con la "mezcla D/D". Los dos componentes principales, el 1,3-dicloropropeno y el 1,2-

dicloropropano, se eliminan con rapidez, principalmente por la orina y, en menor cantidad, por el aire expirado. Los componentes de la "mezcla D/D" se metabolizan por oxidación y conjugación. Los principales metabolitos urinarios son los ácidos mercaptúricos.

1.3 Efectos en los seres vivos del medio ambiente

La "mezcla D/D" es moderadamente tóxica para los peces; los valores de la CL_{50} a las 96 h oscilan entre 1 y 6 mg/litro. La toxicidad de la mezcla se debe fundamentalmente al 1,3-dicloropropeno.

Cuando se utilizan las dosis de aplicación recomendadas, los principales efectos de la "mezcla D/D" son la reducción transitoria (< 7 días) de los hongos del suelo y la inhibición de la oxidación de los iones amonio a nitrato. La mezcla es tóxica para las bacterias nitrificantes. Inmediatamente después de desaparecer del suelo, las bacterias comienzan a colonizar la zona de nuevo. En ensayos de campo, la "mezcla D/D" (aplicada a 600 litros/ha) eliminó los invertebrados del suelo. La recolonización requirió entre 6 y 24 meses.

La "mezcla D/D" tiene una elevada fitotoxicidad.

1.4 Efectos en los animales de experimentación y en sistemas de prueba in vitro

La toxicidad aguda de la "mezcla D/D" para los animales de laboratorio es de moderada a alta. Los valores de la DL_{50} por vía oral en ratas y ratones oscilan entre 132 y 300 mg/kg de peso corporal. Los valores de la DL_{50} por vía cutánea en ratas y conejos son de 779 y 2100 mg/kg de peso corporal, respectivamente. La CL_{50} (4 h) por vía respiratoria para ratas es aproximadamente de 4540 mg/m^3. La exposición aguda produjo signos clínicos asociados a depresión del sistema nervioso central. La "mezcla D/D" tiene un fuerte efecto irritante en los ojos y la piel y una moderada capacidad de sensibilización cutánea.

Los resultados de los estudios disponibles de toxicidad durante un período breve en ratas y perros son insuficientes para evaluar de manera correcta la posible toxicidad de la mezcla, porque las dosis relativamente bajas ensayadas no demuestran ningún efecto biológicamente significativo. Se han realizado varios estudios de exposición por inhalación (todo el cuerpo) durante un período corto en ratas. Las concentraciones de hasta 145 mg/m^3 de la "mezcla D/D" no tienen ningún efecto tóxico. Con niveles de 1362 mg/m^3 o superiores se detectan claramente efectos tóxicos asociados con depresión del sistema nervioso central. Una exposición a 443 mg/m^3 durante 10 semanas da lugar a una disminución del aumento del peso corporal y a un mayor peso absoluto de los riñones.

Un estudio teratológico en ratas por vía oral de la "mezcla D/D" fue inadecuado para evaluar su posible acción en este sentido.

En un estudio de inhalación en ratas con dosis de hasta 443 mg/m^3 durante 10 semanas, para investigar la fecundidad de machos y hembras, no se observó ningún efecto. Debido a un diseño inadecuado del procedimiento, no fue posible evaluar completamente los efectos de la "mezcla D/D" sobre la reproducción.

La mezcla tiene efectos mutagénicos en las cepas TA100 y TA1535 de *Salmonella typhimurium*, así como en la WP2 HCR de *Escherichia coli*, sin activación metabólica. Sin embargo, no se produjeron tales efectos en las cepas TA98, TA1537 y TA1538 de *Salmonella*.

En un estudio prolongado en ratas alimentadas con dietas que contenían hasta 120 mg de la "mezcla D/D" por kg (equivalentes a 6 mg/kg de peso corporal) durante dos años no se detectaron efectos tóxicos ni carcinógenos.

1.5 Efectos en el ser humano

Ya no se utiliza la "mezcla D/D" tanto como antes, por lo que es improbable la exposición de la población general a través del aire, el agua y los alimentos.

Cuando se utilizaban los procedimientos recomendados, la exposición de los trabajadores que llenaban los bidones y de los aplicadores en el campo fue en general inferior a 4,5 mg de 1,3-dicloropropeno/m^3. En otras condiciones se han medido concentraciones de hasta 36,32 mg/m^3.

Se ha informado de un caso de intoxicación aguda con desenlace fatal tras la ingestión accidental de la mezcla.

Se han notificado varios casos de dermatitis por contacto y de sensibilización cutánea debidas a la exposición accidental a la "mezcla D/D".

2. Conclusiones

- Población general: Dado que la "mezcla D/D" no tiene ya un uso tan generalizado, la exposición de la población al 1,3-dicloropropeno a través del aire, el agua y los alimentos es insignificante, pero, en ciertas zonas, cuando se contaminan las aguas subterráneas, se puede producir una exposición al 1,2-dicloropropano.

- Exposición profesional: Durante las actividades de llenado y de aplicación de la "mezcla D/D" en los campos se puede producir una exposición de los manipuladores a concentraciones de 1,3-dicloropropeno superiores a la máxima permisible, especialmente en condiciones climáticas cálidas.

- Medio ambiente: No es probable que la "mezcla D/D" alcance niveles biológicamente significativos en el medio terrestre o acuático, siempre que se utilice en las dosis recomendadas. Tampoco es probable que se produzcan efectos adversos duraderos en los organismos vivos del medio ambiente.

3. Recomendaciones

- No se debe utilizar la "mezcla D/D" para fumigar el suelo, debido a su capacidad de lixiviar y alcanzar las aguas subterráneas.

- En las zonas en las que se use la mezcla, se han de vigilar los residuos en las aguas superficiales y subterráneas.

www.ingramcontent.com/pod-product-compliance
Ingram Content Group UK Ltd.
Pitfield, Milton Keynes, MK11 3LW, UK
UKHW021314180426
11947UKWH00015B/1214